Esophageal Cancer Surgery

T0332369

A specialist clinical monograph for thoracic and general surgeons who specialize in the treatment of esophageal cancer, supported by practical images and video.

Esophageal cancer is a challenging area which includes the specialties of gastro-hepatology, radiology, radio-chemotherapy, anesthesia, psychology, and surgery, requiring treatment by a multidisciplinary team. In this type of surgery tumors located in the middle and upper one-third present a particular challenge, so the author describes how the use of the Akiyama procedure can alleviate this, maximizing operative access.

This content is suitable for practicing surgeons with a range of surgical experience, and the step-by-step approach is fully illustrated with both photographs and access to operative videos. Key points are described, and potential pitfalls explained.

Henri Kolani is Associate Professor of Surgery and Consultant General Surgeon at the Mother Theresa University Hospital Center in Tirana, Albania. The hospital has a capacity of 1,612 beds and employs more than 2,500 people. Dr. Kolani has the wide-ranging surgical experience of a general surgeon, but has specialized in surgical oncology, and, in particular, pancreato-hepatobiliary and eso-gastric surgery, performing classical-style major oncological surgeries.

Esophageal Cancer Surgery
Surgery
Akiyama Procedure

Henri Kolani

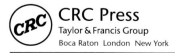

CRC Press
Taylor & Francis Group
Boca Raton London New York

CRC Press is an imprint of the
Taylor & Francis Group, an **informa** business

First edition published 2025
by CRC Press
2385 NW Executive Center Drive, Suite 320, Boca Raton FL 33431

and by CRC Press
4 Park Square, Milton Park, Abingdon, Oxon, OX14 4RN

CRC Press is an imprint of Taylor & Francis Group, LLC

© 2025 Henri Kolani

This book contains information obtained from authentic and highly regarded sources. While all reasonable efforts have been made to publish reliable data and information, neither the author[s] nor the publisher can accept any legal responsibility or liability for any errors or omissions that may be made. The publishers wish to make clear that any views or opinions expressed in this book by individual editors, authors or contributors are personal to them and do not necessarily reflect the views/opinions of the publishers. The information or guidance contained in this book is intended for use by medical, scientific or health-care professionals and is provided strictly as a supplement to the medical or other professional's own judgement, their knowledge of the patient's medical history, relevant manufacturer's instructions and the appropriate best practice guidelines. Because of the rapid advances in medical science, any information or advice on dosages, procedures or diagnoses should be independently verified. The reader is strongly urged to consult the relevant national drug formulary and the drug companies' and device or material manufacturers' printed instructions, and their websites, before administering or utilizing any of the drugs, devices or materials mentioned in this book. This book does not indicate whether a particular treatment is appropriate or suitable for a particular individual. Ultimately it is the sole responsibility of the medical professional to make his or her own professional judgements, so as to advise and treat patients appropriately. The authors and publishers have also attempted to trace the copyright holders of all material reproduced in this publication and apologize to copyright holders if permission to publish in this form has not been obtained. If any copyright material has not been acknowledged please write and let us know so we may rectify in any future reprint.

ISBN: 978-1-032-80586-3 (hbk)
ISBN: 978-1-032-80582-5 (pbk)
ISBN: 978-1-003-49754-7 (ebk)

DOI: 10.1201/9781003497547

Typeset in Sabon
by Apex CoVantage, LLC

I dedicate this monograph to my entire family. A special honor in the memory of my father Lika, my mother Margarita, my brother Robert who I find inspiring in every time and situation. I thank my sister Urana, Maksim and Kristian for the support in my profession.

A special thanks to my wife Evis and my twin sons Franc and Robert for their constant inspiration, understanding, tolerance and encouragement in my career.

Contents

Video List

Access to surgical videos demonstrating surgical techniques is available via QR code.

(www.youtube.com/@HenriKolani/videos)

Surgical Techniques

- Akiyama Procedure—Summary of Four Cases of Esophageal Cancer
- Akiyama Procedure—Full Video of Fifth Case of Esophageal Cancer
- Left Hepatectomy Reglee for Cholangiocarcinoma
- Classic Blumgart: Pancreatico-Jejunostomy in Whipple Procedure
- Pancreatico-Jejunostomy with Stent, Blumgart procedure. Whipple Procedure Plus Right Hemicolectomy
- Morbus Caroli: Partial Hepatic Resection; Hepatico-Jejunostomy in Roux-en-Y
- Distal Esophagectomy. Ivor-Lewis Procedure. Right Toracotomy
- Distal Esophagectomy. Left Thoracotomy. Procedure Ivor-Lewis
- Right Hepatectomy Reglee for Hepatocarcinoma
- Resection of the Body and Tail of the Pancreas
- Pancreaticoduodenectomy. Whipple Procedure
- Retroperitoneal Formation Attached to the Vena Cava
- Akiyama Procedure. Thoracic Phase. Part I
- Akiyama Procedure. Abdominal Phase. Part II
- Retroperitoneal Subhepatic Formation
- Esophagectomy. Akiyama Procedure. Cervical Phase. Part III
- Extirpation of the Tumor Formation, Left Nephrectomy and Right Left Adrenalectomy En Bloc
- Surgical Treatment of Rectocele
- Vaginal and Perianal Condyloma

- Akiyama Procedure. Full Video of the Sixth Case of Esophageal Cancer
- Akiyama Procedure. Retrosternal Tunnel Preparation and Stomach Transposition
- Akiyama Procedure. Subtotal Esophagectomy. Abdominal Phase
- Subtotal Esophagectomy. Akiyama Procedure. Cervical Stage
- Subtotal Esophagectomy. Akiyama Procedure. Thoracic Phase
- Akiyama Procedure. Gastric Tube Preparation

Preface

In order to achieve a high-quality surgery, a good knowledge of anatomy and the correct implementation of operative techniques are of great importance.

Progress in esophageal surgery depends on experience in patient care, accurate data collection, the surgeon's performance, and effective and honest reporting of results to the surgical community. In surgery in general, and that of the esophagus in particular, the complications begin with the surgeon and the success or failure of the patient ends with the surgeon.

All surgeons, in the postoperative period, know very well the weak point in the intervention they performed, but they are not happy to accept it. Therefore, great care is needed in all steps of the intervention, because a small negligence that at first glance seems insignificant can complicate the intervention and be fatal. Catching the complication as soon as possible and taking active action to correct it is vital for the patient.

Nowadays, there is no room for invention in this field of surgery, as all the procedures have been done and explained very clearly in various treatises, but the meticulous implementation of all operative moments remains the duty of every surgeon, especially of the young surgeons, the contingent I, too, am part of.

I cannot refrain from mentioning Professor Besim Elezi, the pioneer surgeon of this difficult part of the esophagus, the upper one-third of it. I studied with care and attention all the records of the esophageal surgeries of Professor Elezi, with lesions in the upper one-third, both neoplasia and burns of the esophagus, where a great help was given by the statistical center at QSUT and in Durres, where the professor continued his activity. In all cases, the professor explains clearly, precisely, and professionally the use of the colon to replace the resected esophagus. These are a great source of educational material and help for any surgeon. This gave me a strong indication to try using the stomach to replace the esophagus, as a more physiological alternative with fewer complications.

We should not be discouraged by the fact that innovations are in most cases met with envy and skepticism. On the contrary, we should work even harder to achieve quality and coherence in this type of surgery. The very first case of the Akiyama procedure with cervical eso-gastro anastomosis that I performed was labeled as an experiment, despite the fact that the world has been doing it since 1976. I have been dealing with esophageal surgery for over a decade, a surgery as complex as it is, which requires multidisciplinary treatment, including radiotherapy, chemotherapy, and surgery. The patient's life is extended, however, when surgical treatment is provided.

In this monograph I have displayed my personal experience for the last five years. I initiated treatment with the Ivor-Lewis technique for tumors located in the lower one-third of the esophagus. Subsequently, we accomplished the Akiyama procedure for the first time to address pathologies affecting the upper and middle one-third of the esophagus. Let me clarify—I performed the Akiyama procedure for the first time in Albania with the interposition of the retrosternal gastric tube and cervical eso-gastric anastomosis, as this procedure had been performed before in the country, but in all cases the transverse colon is used as a substitute for the esophagus. The innovation I brought is the stomach as a replacement, which is described in this monograph, both with the operative technique and its secrets: showing where the stomach incision begins, how it continues, the width of the gastric tube, the making and expansion of the retrosternal tunnel, fixing of the stomach so that it does not twist. And all these secrets are described to be easily practiced by my fellow surgeons. If I have given my thoughts on why I have chosen the Akiyama procedure, why a right thoracotomy, the role of preoperative radio-chemotherapy, the role of feeding jejunostomy, complications, and postoperative results. Based on the tumor's location within the esophagus and the need to maintain an appropriate oncological margin when dividing the normal esophagus above the tumor's border, I believe it is necessary to surgically separate the esophagus into two distinct sections: (1) the lower portion where the Ivor-Lewis procedure should be performed and (2) the upper and middle portion, for which the Akiyama or McKeown procedure should be performed. This is still up for debate.

I have carried the glory of success and the shame of defeat on my shoulders.

I am of the opinion that we should not get carried away by the mania to perform major surgery. In cases with carcinoma of the esophagus, we must not always stick strictly to the established protocol, but in special cases we must step out of the "line", selecting the strategy and type of intervention in accordance with the clinical conditions of the patient, which are individual, in order to reduce complications and most importantly to improve the quality of his life.

The choice between a neck or thoracic anastomosis remains a topic of ongoing debate within the surgical community. It seems that the personal preferences and expertise of individual surgeons may carry greater significance than the specific method selected for anastomosis.

All patients who will be selected to perform an esophageal resection procedure must first undergo the placement of a feeding jejunostomy or esophageal stent, then continue with full radiotherapy sessions and three to four cycles of chemotherapy. After these steps, we come to the final one, resection of the esophagus. In most cases, I have performed right or left thoracotomy because I have paid special attention to lymphatic drainage in the face of a malignant pathology, and despite conflicting opinions, for me, lymphatic drainage affects the prolongation of survival. But can we perform a radical lymphatic curage in all cases with carcinoma of the esophagus? I have given my opinion below on this question as well. In a few cases, I performed distal transhiatal esophagectomy, since the tumor was located in the lower one-third of the esophagus, that is, superior polar resection.

However, we have a small population in number compared to large countries such as China, Japan, etc., therefore the number of cases are limited and the results and opinions are modest, but the desire to work is great. These cases and the results that I have described in this monograph are easily verifiable in the statistical center, in the collective of surgeons where I work at the Mother Theresa University Hospital Center, with respected and affirmed professors in this field of surgery in Albania, in the Ministry of Health as it has promoted my work, as well as in the photos and videos of the operations that I have done, a good part of which I have presented in this monograph. I feel lucky that I was able to perform Nine cases with the Akiyama procedure, because you can work all your life as a surgeon and may not be able to perform it again, because the cases are presented at an advanced stage of carcinoma that is inoperable.

I want to extend my heartfelt thanks and deep gratitude to my teachers, professors, specialist physicians, the entire clinical team, medical practitioners, gastro-hepatologists, anatomopathologists, laboratory technicians, and the dedicated personnel in the resuscitation department who have played a pivotal role in shaping my professional journey and contributing to my success. Special thanks to the imaging doctor Dr. Renato Perlat Osmënaj, for the great contribution he has given us in this contingent of patients. Many thanks to Miranda Bromage, Greig Hudson, Kate Fornadel, and all associated Taylor & Francis staff, for their help and effort in making this work have a wider, global outreach.

I express my gratitude to Professor Albana Fico, the General Director of Mother Teresa University Hospital Tirana, for her unwavering support to the implementation of best standards of care and medical innovation.

I thank Professor Stefan Jianu, whose student I am and Professor Sorin Paun for the long consultations and the input they gave me before I realized the first case with the Akiyama procedure.

A man is not born a surgeon, he becomes one through work, but the desire and passion for surgery ends with the departure of his soul.

Henri Kolani

Author

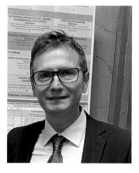 **Henri Kolani** was born June 8, 1971, to a prominent family in Berat. His father, Lika Kolani, was a WWII veteran and a renowned pharmacist who graduated in Budapest. His mother, Margarita, was a professor of English language and the niece of Lasgush Poradeci.

In 1994, he graduated as a general physician from the Faculty of Medicine, University of Tirana.

From 1996 to 2001 he completed the cycle of full long-term specialization in general surgery at Spitalul Clinic de Urgenta Floreasca Bucuresti.

In 2001, he graduated as a general surgeon from the Carol Davila University of Medicine and Pharmacy in Bucharest.

From 2002 he worked as a surgeon at the Mother Teresa University Hospital Center in Tirana.

From 2011 onward Dr. Kolani has been a professor and head of Surgical Semiotics in the faculty of dental medicine at Tirana University of Medicine.

In 2016, he defended his scientific degree, Doctor of Science, given by the faculty of medicine, University of Medicine Tirana.

He has completed several short-term specializations in EU countries in digestive surgery, especially in surgery of the liver, pancreas, and esophageal surgery.

Dr. Kolani is a member of various surgical boards and associations at home and abroad, as well as a full member of The International Society of University Colon and Rectal Surgeons, King's College in London, England.

He speaks three languages: Romanian, English, and Italian.

He has published many articles in scientific journals with an impact factor, both within and outside the country.

In 2020, in Germany, he published a monograph entitled *Current Approach of Surgical Technique of Upper and Lower Colo-Rectal Anastomosis, Early and Late Complications*.

In 2021, he defended his scientific degree, Associated Professor, given by the faculty of medicine at the University of Medicine in Tirana, approved by the Albanian Ministry of Education.

Chapter 1

A Brief History of Esophageal Surgery

An important role in the renaissance of esophageal surgery has been played by the advancement of anesthesia. Advances in the surgery of benign diseases led to the development of surgery for malignant diseases, but in esophageal surgery the improvement came simultaneously for both benign and malignant diseases.

German clinician Adolf Kussmaul performed the first esophagoscopy in 1868.

In 1877 Vincenz Czerny performed the resection of a carcinoma of the cervical esophagus without restoring the esophageal transit.

In 1879 the great Theodor Billtoth resected a carcinoma of the esophagus en bloc with the larynx and thyroid gland.

In 1909, Evans performed the first resection of carcinoma of the esophagus and restored transit with an external rubber tube.

The first to perform transthoracic esophagectomy was Franz Torek in 1913.

In 1913 Johannes Zaaijer in the Netherlands performed a transpleural resection of a carcinoma in the lower one-third of the esophagus.

Oshawa from Kyoto, Japan in 1933 performed the first transthoracic esophagectomy and esophagogastrostomy in nine stages.

In England in 1933 Gray Turner performed the first transhiatal esophagectomy.

Hiroshi Akiyama from Tokyo performed the hypopharyngeal resection.

In 1976 McKeown from Darlington performed the esophagectomy with neck anastomosis.

In the United States the surgeon Orringer popularized the transhiatal resection. In Japan, special importance is attached to detailed lymphatic curage.

Alfred Cuschieri from Dundee performed the first thoracic esophagectomy with a thoracoscope in 1992.

Currently, the total MIE performed by Jim Luketich of Pittsburgh is becoming the standard surgical treatment.

DOI: 10.1201/9781003497547-1

Esophageal surgery, too, has had a progressive evolution in Albania. As the pioneers of this surgery, we can mention Professor Petro Cani and Professor Besim Elezi, followed by Professor Nikollaq Kaçani, Professor Etmont Çeliku, Professor Arben Gjata, and Professor Arben Beqiri. Notably, Professor Besim Elezi, during his career dedicated an important part to the cervical esophagus surgery, as one of the most difficult fields of the profession. After performing subtotal esophageal resection, he achieved the replacement of the esophagus with a part of colon, thus giving a solution and a great help to the patients (information from the database of the Statistics Center of Mother Teresa University Hospital, as well from the most recent interview of Professor Besim Elezi during a TV show "Magic of the Scalpel" on Albanian National Radio Television, March 2023.

BIBLIOGRAPHY

Qian ZX. Investigation on esophageal cancer in the province of Xinjiang: Collected papers of the second symposium on esophageal carcinoma. Chin Acad Med Sci. 1961:74–8.

Kühn CG, editor. De symptomatum causis. In: Claudii Galeni opera omnia. Tom VII, pars L. Leipzig: Knoblosh; 1824.

Karamanou M, Tsoucalas G, Saridaki Z, et al. Avenzoar's (1091–1162) clinical description of cancer. J BUON. 2015;20:1171–4.

Vesalius A. The fabric of the human body. In: Garrison DH, Hast MH, editors. An annotated translation of the 1543 and 1555 editions of "De Humanic Corporis Fabrica Libri Septem". Book 5. vol. 2. Karger; 2014. p. 948 and 990.

Fernel J. De Morbis Universalibus et Particularibus. libri IV posteriores pathologiae. Paris: Hieronymum Blageart; 1645.

Bonet T. Sepulchretum sive anatomia practica. Geneva: Chouet; 1700.

Robinson DH, Toledo AH. Historical development of modern anesthesia. J Invest Surg. 2012;25:141–9. doi: 10.3109/08941939.2012.690328.

Earrington B, Vesalius A. The last chapter of the De Fabrica of Vesalius entitled some observations on the dissection of living animals. Latin Trans Roy Soc S Africa. 1931;20:1–14. doi: 10.1080/00359193109518843.

Sauerbruch F. Zur Pathologie des offenen Pneumothorax und die Grundlagen meines-Verfahrens zu seiner Ausschaltung. Mitteil Grenzgeb Med Chir. 1904;13:399–482.

Brauer L. Die Ausschaltung der Pneumothoraxfolgen mit Hilfe des Ueberdruckverfahrens. Mitteil Grenzgeb Med Chir. 1904;13:483–500.

Meltzer SJ, Auer J. Continuous respiration without respiratory movements. J Exp Med. 1909;11:622–5. doi: 10.1084/jem.11.4.622.

Guedel AE, Waters RM. A new intra-tracheal catheter. Anesth Analg. 1928;7:238–9. doi: 10.1213/00000539-192801000-00089.

Gale J, Waters M. Closed endobronchial anaesthesia in thoracic surgery. J Thorac Surg. 1932;1:432–7. doi: 10.1016/S0096-5588(20)32547-2.

Rowbotham S. Laryngeal intubation in anesthetics. Br Med J. 1923;1:1090–1. doi: 10.1136/bmj.1.3261.1090.

Magill W. Endotracheal anesthesia. Proc R Soc Med. 1928;22:83–8. doi: 10.1177/003591572802200201.

Carlens E. A new flexible double-lumen catheter for bronchospirometry. J Thorac Surg. 1949;18:742–6. doi: 10.1016/S0096-5588(20)31326-X.

Robertshaw FL. Low resistance double-lumen endobronchial tubes. Br J Anaesth. 1962;34:576–9. doi: 10.1093/bja/34.8.576.

Kacmarek RM. The mechanical ventilator: Past, present, and future. Respir Care. 2011;56:1170–80. doi: 10.4187/respcare.01420.

Kussmaul A. Zur geschichte der oesophago und gastroskopie. Arch Klin Med. 1898;6:456.

Czerny V. Neue operationen. Zentralbl Chir. 1877;4:433–4.

Karamanou M, Markatos K, Lymperi M, et al. A historical overview of laryngeal carcinoma and the first total laryngectomies. J BUON. 2017;22:807–11.

Billroth CAT. Totalextirpation des Ganzenoesophagus vom Pharynx bis zum Sternum; ein Totalextirpation des Ganzenlarynx mit des ganzen Schilddruse. Verhandl Deut Ges Chir. 1879;8:7–9.

Mikulicz J, von. Ein Fall von Resektion des Carcinomatosen Oesophagus mit plastichen Ersatz des exeidirten Stuckes. Prag Med Wochenschr. 1886;11:93–4.

Evans A. Rubber esophagus. Br J Surg. 1932;20:388–92. doi: 10.1002/bjs.1800207904.

Edwards AT. Transpleural removal of total thoracic oesophagus. Proc R Soc Med. 1935;29:188–90. doi: 10.1177/003591573502900230.

Dobromysslov WD. Ein Fall von transpleuraler Osophagotomie im Brustabschnitte. Zbl Chir. 1901;1:18.

Meade R. A history of thoracic surgery. Springfield, (IL, USA): Charles C Thomas; 1961. p. 662.

Torek F. The first successful resection of the thoracic portion of the esophagus for carcinoma. Surg Gyn Obstet. 1913;16:614–17. doi: 10.1001/jama.1913.04340200023008.

Eggers C. Resection of the thoracic portion of the esophagus for carcinoma. Arch Surg. 1925:10:361–73. doi: 10.1001/archsurg.1925.01120100373020.

Zaaijer JH. Erfolgreiche transpleurale Resektion eines Cardiacarcinomas. Beitr Klin Chir. 1913;83:419–22.

von Ach A. Beiträge zur ösophagus-chirurgie [dissertation]. Munich, Germany: J.F. Lehmann's Verlag; 1913.

Denk W. Zur Radikaloperation des Oesophaguskarzinoms (vorläufige Mittelung). Zentralbl Chir. 1913;40:1065–8.

Ohsawa T. Esophageal surgery. Nippon Geka Gakkai Zasshi. 1933;34:1318–590.

Marshall SF. Carcinoma of the esophagus: Successful resection of lower end of oesophagus with re-establishment of esophageal gastric continuity. Surg Clin North Am. 1938;18:643–8.

Adams W, Phemister DB. Carcinoma of the lower thoracic esophagus: Report of a successful resection and esophago-gastrostomy. J Thorac Surg. 1938;7:621–7. doi: 10.1016/S0096-5588(20)32131-0.

Wu YK, Loucks HH. Surgical treatment of carcinoma of the esophagus. Chin Med J. 1941;60:1–33.

Thompson VC. Carcinoma of the oesophagus: Resection and oesophago-gastrostomy. Br J Surg. 1945;32:377–80. doi: 10.1002/bjs.18003212707.

Chapter 2

Embryology, Anatomy, and Physiology of Esophagus

2.1 EMBRYOLOGY

A deviation of the anterior intestine almost on the 22nd gestational day leads to the formation of the esophagus, which follows a path from the respiratory diverticulum to the fusiform one, the end side of which gives the formation of the stomach.

The development of the lateral crests of the proliferating epithelium in the fifth gestational week leads to the separation of the trachea from the esophagus by dividing its lumen into an anterior and a posterior part. This division is a provisional division and is represented by the tracheo-esophageal septum. The final separation of the esophagus and trachea occurs in the 36th week and is achieved through the necrosis of the formed septa. When this process is not well carried out, it leads to the formation of various anomalies such as esophago-tracheal fistula.

The length of the esophagus at this stage is approximately 2.5 mm and as the days go by it enlarges, reaching a length of 5 mm on the 32nd day. Its extension continues until the end of the seventh week where it reaches its maximum length. Any alteration in this process can lead to the formation of the pathology of esophageal atresia.

The lumen of the esophagus is obliterated around the seventh week, through the process of columnar cell proliferation.

Between seven and eight weeks, some extracellular vacuoles are formed, between the epithelial cells, at the moment when the lumen of the esophagus thickens. These vacuoles are separated from each other and from the lumen of the esophagus itself by several thin epithelial septa. Further, in weeks 11 to 12, the process of vacuolization takes place, which consists in the fusion, union, and disappearance of the aforementioned vacuoles. Cysts and other abnormalities such as duplication of the esophagus are the explanation that this process has not been carried out correctly. Despite the aforementioned, different authors debate these facts, because

DOI: 10.1201/9781003497547-2

they are of the opinion that it is the irregularity in epithelial proliferation that forms epithelial bridges represented by vacuoles.

From the eighth week, a predominance of ciliary cells compared to columnar ones is observed, also at this time we have the evidence of non-ciliary cells and goblets. Some authors are of the opinion that mucin-positive globular cells become more numerous during the fourth month, and during this time, the process of cell degeneration and stratification persists. Squamous cells are evident in the middle esophagus during the fifth to sixth months; the process extends in two directions, proximal and distal, replacing mucin-secreting ciliated cells. At the same time, in the upper esophagus we can have columnar cells, which can be surrounded by islet-shaped secretory cells. These secretory cells are called cardiac glands and are superficial to the muscularis mucosa. On the other hand, the deep submucosa is poor in secretory and parietal cells, which develop later than the seventh month.

Supportive tissues, musculature and vascularization, are of mesodermal origin.

The muscles of the esophagus are of mesenchymal origin, namely in the upper two-thirds of the esophagus the striated musculature originates from the mesenchyme of the brachial arch, while in the lower one-third the smooth muscle originates from the splanchnic mesenchyme. Based on what was said above, where the mesenchymal origin was stated, abnormalities in the development of the aortic arch can also lead to problems or abnormalities in the esophageal development, also causing cases of dysphagia such as "Luzoria Dysphagia", where the right subclavian artery follows a path behind the esophagus. The muscularis propria layer and its musculature are seen after the sixth week.

Characteristic is the presence of smooth musculature of the esophagus throughout its length, though striated musculature is present in the somatic musculature.

Following the ninth week of development, striated muscle fibers become apparent in the upper segment of the muscularis propria. This striation continues throughout the entire length of the esophagus until approximately the fifth month of development, predominantly in the upper one-third of the esophageal muscles. During the initial phases of esophageal development, neuroblasts emerge at the outer edges of the circular musculature, ultimately forming complete rings in conjunction with the myenteric and submucosal plexuses.

2.2 ANATOMY

The esophagus has two characteristics: it is elastic and contractible. It is described as a membranous-muscular tube with a length of 25 cm and a diameter of 2 cm and performs well the function of passing the food bolus toward the stomach.

The upper termination point of the inferior laryngeal nerve is within the inferior constrictor muscle of the pharynx. On the other hand, the lower extent of the esophagus is marked by the cardia, which serves as the transition point from the esophagus to the stomach.

During its journey in the thorax, the esophagus makes an inflection at the level of the fourth thoracic vertebra, following a progressive trajectory away from the vertebrae. The portions of the esophagus are divided in correspondence to the path that it follows, namely it is divided into three regions, the cervical, thoracic, and abdominal esophagus. In daily practice using endoscopy as a tool, the superior end of the esophagus begins at the dental arcade, which is located 15 cm from the pharyngo-esophageal junction.

The cervical portion of the esophagus starts from the sixth cervical vertebra to the first thoracic vertebra, with a length of 6 cm. In this portion we have the presence of the lower esophageal sphincter, which is formed by the combination of the circular fibers of the smooth muscle with the fibers of the inferior constrictor and cricopharyngeal muscles.

The portion of the thoracic esophagus has a length of 15–16 cm and follows a path from the first thoracic vertebra to the 11th thoracic vertebra.

The penetration of the diaphragm from the esophagus at the level of the tenth thoracic vertebra constitutes the portion of the diaphragmatic esophagus.

The abdominal portion of the esophagus constitutes its final part. As we mentioned before, its final edge considering it as a single entity was 40 cm from the incisors. With a length of 3–4 cm, it is easily detected by the endoscope at a length of 36–40 cm from the incisors. Nowadays the notion of a higher-pressure area in the terminal part of the esophagus refutes what for many years was known as nosology, the lower esophageal sphincter. In terms of appearance, the esophagus, in its superior portion, takes on an antero-posterior compressed shape, and three areas of narrowing are evident:

1) *The first constriction*, Cricopharyngeal, with a length of 1.5 cm and a diameter of 1.6 cm, which in terms of dimensions is the shortest and narrowest portion.
2) *The second narrowing*, the aorto-bronchial one, with a length of 5 cm and a diameter of 1.7 cm, has an extension from the fourth thoracic vertebra to the fifth thoracic vertebra. This narrowing is attributed to the contact of the esophagus with the aorta and left bronchus.
3) *The third constriction*, occurs at the level of the diaphragmatic passage, has a length of 1–2 cm and a diameter of about 1.9 cm.

Based on the explanation of these three narrowings, the esophagus is divided into three segments, the subdiaphragmatic, broncho-diaphragmatic, and crico-aortic.

2.2.1 The Structure of the Esophageal Wall

The esophageal mucosa is formed by three layers, the color of which in the endoscopic examination is light pink.

The oropharyngeal mucosa continues with stratified squamous epithelium, and beneath this epithelium lies an acellular layer called the lamina propria, which is rich in a network of mucinous glands and also a network of blood and lymphatic vessels. Beneath it, with a longitudinal arrangement and formed by smooth muscle, lies the muscularis mucosae layer, which is also the strongest layer of the esophagus wall.

Endoscopically, the transition of the light pink esophageal mucosa to the reddish-pink gastric mucosa is represented by Linea Z, but this border is not defined as the inferior anatomic border.

The submucosa represents an aspect of the connective tissue which is characterized by the presence of arterial, venous, lymphatic plexuses, Meissner's plexus, and elastic fibers.

The easy passage of food from the esophagus to the stomach is achieved by the mucosal and submucosal glands, which in turn provide a lubricating layer.

The muscular layer is composed of an inner layer of circular muscles and an outer layer of longitudinal muscles, with the myenteric ganglia of Auerbach and Meissner situated between them. The muscular layer along the entire path of the esophagus is divided into three portions and has special characteristics for each division. In the upper one-third, voluntary striated muscle predominates, in the middle one-third, voluntary striated muscle is combined with involuntary smooth muscle and in the last portion of the lower one-third, only smooth muscle predominates. It is precisely this construction which mediates the passage of food into the stomach without the need for the exercise of force by the striated muscles. The time for the passage of the food bolus from the oral to the esophageal cavity is mediated by the upper esophageal sphincter. The function of which is to keep the esophagus closed and open only during the swallowing process.

Its composition we can mention the posterior part of the cricoid and thyroid cartilage, the hyoid bone and three muscles, the cricopharyngeal, inferior thyropharyngeal constrictor, and the cranial part of the cervical esophagus. The combination of the aforementioned muscles form a triangle called the Kilian triangle, an area in which we often encounter Zenker's diverticula.

The thyro-esophageal muscle is primarily made up of muscular tissue, whereas the cricothyroid muscle consists of a combination of slow and fast muscle fibers, the prevalence of which depends on whether they are located in the pharyngeal or esophageal region. In the cranial part of the pharynx, slow fibers are predominantly found, and as they descend caudally, they merge with the circular musculature of the esophagus. Next, the food bolus, after crossing the entire esophageal track, reaches the lower sphincter, which opens to pass the food and then closes again to prevent food regurgitation and gastro-esophageal reflux. The two components for the proper functioning of the sphincter are:

1) *High pressure area*, which responds to changes in intra-abdominal pressures.
2) *The component of the diaphragmatic muscle*, from the esophagus passage through the diaphragm, it can serve as another sphincter, increasing the pressure in the distal esophagus, in relation to the respiratory process.

The normal functioning of the esophagus is achieved by its four composing layers:

1) *The mucosal layer* is the inner layer of the esophagus, which is characterized by the presence of the majority of glands that produce mucus, and non-keratinized epithelial cells. Since it is the inner layer of the esophagus, it has direct contact with the food that passes through it, and the cells in this layer best perform lubrication and protection of this organ from stomach acid, from solid foods, and it is the only layer that has direct contact with the compounds that pass along this organ.
2) Below the mucosal layer comes *the submucosa*, which is traversed by blood vessels that supply the mucosal layer and is rich in connective tissue.
3) *The muscular layer*, consisting of striated and smooth muscles, is responsible for peristalsis of the esophagus, directing the food bolus from the oral cavity toward the stomach. The skeletal musculature of the esophagus following the longitudinal direction is organized into three muscle fascicles.

Two of these fascicles are described as continuations of the pharyngeal musculature, while the first fascicle is fixed to the posterior aspect of the cricoid cartilage via the crico-esophageal ligament. In continuation, the three fascicles descending downward form a uniform surface which wraps the esophagus.

The circular muscle fibers responsible for facilitating the passage of the food bolus from the esophagus to the stomach have their origin as an extension of the constrictor muscle in the hypopharynx. They are arranged transversely in both the upper and lower regions of the esophagus and follow an oblique orientation along the body of the esophagus. It is worth noting that the outer muscle layer is thinner than the inner one, and besides this fact, immediately after exiting the diaphragm, the muscle layer begins to thicken, the muscle fibers at this level become semicircular, fusing with the muscles of the lower esophageal sphincter.

4) The last layer is *the adventitia*, which ensures the fixation of the esophagus and other organs and wraps the muscular layer of the esophagus.

The esophagus has no serous lining; however, the connective tissue of the mediastinum gives it a slight adventitial plane, giving the esophagus a degree of motion during deglutition, but when it comes to suture placement, it does not present a clear surgical plane.

2.2.2   Esophageal Reports

2.2.2.1   Cervical Esophagus

The cervical esophagus begins with the pharyngo-esophageal junction which is projected at the level of the sixth cervical vertebra and continues up to the superior border of the thorax which is projected at the level of the first thoracic vertebra.

The pharyngo-esophageal junction represents the boundary between the smooth muscle of the esophagus and the striated muscle of the pharynx.

In the posterior view, a rhombus is formed by the fibers of the inferior constrictor muscle of the pharynx. This rhombus forms two triangles as it is divided horizontally by the cricopharyngeal muscle.

1) The superior triangle, as an area with low functional resistance, projects over the cricopharyngeal muscle. This muscle is also considered as the superior esophageal sphincter.
2) The inferior triangle, as an area covered by circular muscle fibers, projects below the cricopharyngeal muscle. It is precisely the presence of circular fibers that explains the absence of pathology in this area, unlike the upper triangle where we often encounter "Zenker's" diverticulum.

The cervical esophagus following the caudal direction, in the posterior mediastinum, is in close relation with the cervical vertebrae.

- Posteriorly, being separated by a layer of cellulo-adipose tissue, it creates relationships with the cervical column and the paravertebral muscles. The dividing layer mentioned above also represents the plan of the cleavage in the surgical aspect.
- Anteriorly, it contacts with the trachea, whose division is realized by a muscular-fibrous layer, which also serves as a cleavage plane in esophageal surgery. From this portion the esophagus is easily displaced to the left, thus the surgical access of the esophagus is more favorable to the left.

Laterally, the relationship continues with the vasculo-nervous fascia of the neck, which is represented by the common carotid artery, the vagus nerve, the jugular vein, and the sympathetic plexus.

The cervico-thoracic transition zone is projected at the level of the first thoracic vertebra, an area where the esophagus takes a left and posterior position. This positioning makes it relate to the trachea anteriorly and laterally to the vasculo-nervous fascia of the neck. In this area, the thoracic duct makes a shift to the left of the esophagus heading toward the subclavio-jugular confluence, a shift which is of great interest at the time of surgical dissection.

2.2.2.2 Thoracic Esophagus

Of great importance in the study of the thoracic esophagus is the surgical aspect of finding the right access that will make the surgeon's work easier as well as for choosing the right surgical technique.

Division of the esophagus into three parts:

2.2.2.2.1 Upper Esophagus

The superior one-third of the thoracic esophagus, with a positioning leaning to the right in part due to the dimensions of the aortic arch. The reports:

- Posteriorly to the vertebral column and in this area the thoracic duct heads to the subclavian vein leaving the posterior part of the esophagus.
- It is separated from the posterior surface of the trachea by the tracheoesophageal muscle in the front. This close anatomical proximity is the reason why esophageal cancer can quickly invade the trachea.

- On the right in relation to the pleura of the right mediastinum, and along the inferior part in this area, the esophagus has contacts with the vagus nerve, which, after passing along the right side of the trachea, is attached to the esophagus. This area represents an important area of lymphonodal stations for the sole fact that Barety lodge is present in this area.
- On the left, there is a relationship with the pleura of the left mediastinum. Of importance is the presence of Poirier's triangle, along which the superior left intercostal vein passes, and also in this area the left recurrent nerve can be seen together with a lymphonodal bundle.

2.2.2.2.2 Middle Esophagus

It corresponds to the middle one-third of the thoracic esophagus, and for the anatomical reports that this portion presents, such as the trachea, bronchus, arch of the aorta, and descending aorta, it is considered one of the most dangerous routes of the esophagus when we are faced with the surgery of this organ.

- Posteriorly, it is in relation to the vertebral column, from which it takes a progressive distancing, due to the course followed by the descending aorta. The thoracic duct, before passing through the angle formed posteriorly to the arch of the aorta and the hemiazygos vein, approaches the esophagus in the superior portion of the middle mediastinum.
- Anteriorly, through the cellular tissue, it is separated with the trachea, the bifurcation of the trachea and further with the left bronchus. It has a relationship with the inter-tracheo-bronchial lymph nodes, this contact which starts below the bifurcation of the trachea and is mentioned as an area that coincides with the presence of the bronchial arteries, which also emit branches supplying this portion.
- On the right, the esophagus has a relation to the arch of the azygos vein, which then flows into the superior vena cava. The relationship with this vein consists of a crossing that the esophagus makes with this arch, which is often sacrificed during the surgical procedure.
- To the left, the very presence of the aorta at this level, as well as the path of the left recurrent nerve accompanied throughout its course with a lymphonodal bundle seems to hug the aorta and attach to the tracheo-esophageal groove, presents difficulties during the surgical procedure.

2.2.2.2.3 Lower Esophagus

- Posteriorly, after the esophagus progressively moves away from the descending aorta, the thoracic duct, and the azygos veins, it takes a position anterior to the aorta, where the two organs are separated through the cellulo-adipose and lymphatic tissue, between which the esophageal arteries also pass.
- Anteriorly it contacts with the pericardium of the left atrium.
- On the right it follows a path between the azygos vein and the pulmonary ligament. This is the area around the esophagus where the vagus nerve makes a twist by positioning itself behind it.
- On the left, the esophagus creates relationships with the pulmonary peduncle, the pulmonary ligament, and the descending aorta. And just under the arch of the aorta, the vagus nerve makes a twist and is positioned anterior to the esophagus.

2.2.2.3 Diaphragmatic Esophagus

The esophageal hiatus, referred to as the muscular orifice, has an oval shape and is formed by the fibers of the right diaphragmatic crus, at the level of the tenth thoracic vertebra. The external esophageal sphincter is formed by two cruces, the right anterior and the left posterior. This is referred to as an intermediate pressure zone, between positive abdominal and negative thoracic pressure.

2.2.2.4 Abdominal Esophagus

It is the portion extending from the esophageal hiatus to the cardias ventriculi. The phreno-esophageal ligament is connected to the superior portion of the esophagus. Anteriorly, it is in relation to the left lobe of the liver and along its entire course it is accompanied by the anterior vagal plexus.

Posteriorly, it is in relation to the aorta, the retroperitoneal tissue, and during its course it is accompanied by the posterior vagal plexus.

On the left it relates to the angle of His and with the left triangular ligament of the liver.

On the right creates relations with the caudate lobe of the liver and the ventricle.

2.2.3 Vascularization of the Esophagus

The esophagus receives a robust blood supply, beginning with the cervical section and the upper esophageal sphincter, which is nourished by the descending plexus formed by branches of the inferior thyroid artery.

Additionally, this part of the esophagus is also vascularized by a descending branch from the left subclavian artery. The thoracic portion of the esophagus is supplied with blood through branches originating from the bronchial arteries and the aorta. Among which we mention: 1) the anterior esophago-tracheal artery originating from the arch of the aorta or from the left bronchial artery, 2) posterior esophago-tracheal artery which originates from the descending aorta and goes to the right side of the esophagus, 3) the small esophageal artery, originating from the descending aorta, projected at the level of the sixth and seventh thoracic vertebra, and 4) the large esophageal artery, originating from the descending aorta with projection at the level of the seventh and eighth thoracic vertebra (see Figure 2.1).

The distal part of the esophagus, as well as its lower sphincter, are supplied with blood via the left phrenic artery and the left gastric artery. The sub-carinal and supra-diaphragmatic segments are considered the areas with less vascularization, and this is the reason why performing anastomosis at these levels is not advised. The rest of the esophagus is

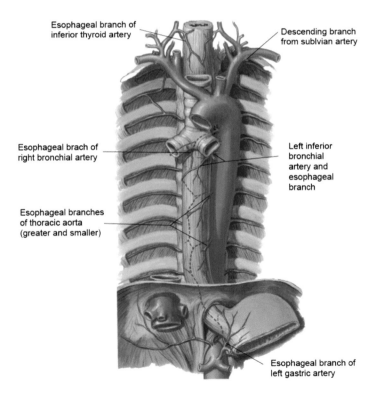

Figure 2.1 **Esophageal arterial system.**

well vascularized, especially from the many branches through which it receives blood supply, which in turn create a dense arterial network in the submucosal layer.

The reason why esophageal infarcts are rare is precisely this arterial network in which numerous anastomosis occur.

Similar to the arterial vascularization, venous drainage is also segmental (see Figure 2.2). The proximal and middle esophageal veins drain into the azygos system, while the superior vena cava is filled by the dense venous plexus. Meanwhile, the distal part of the esophagus drains into a branch of the portal vein or collaterals of the left gastric vein. As from the above, the connection of the distal drainage of the esophagus to the portal system explains the formation of esophageal varices in the case of portal hypertension. Cases of various gastro-intestinal hemorrhages are often attributed to esophageal varices, especially in cases with decompensated hepatic cirrhosis.

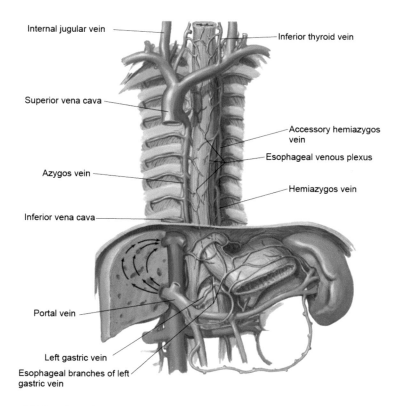

Figure 2.2 Esophageal venous system.

2.2.4   Lymphatic Drainage of the Esophagus

Lymphatic drainage in the esophagus is carried out by lymph nodes and lymphatic channels. The mucosa, submucosa, and muscularis are the levels where the lymphatic channels form lymphatic plexuses (see Figure 2.3). Their beginning in the tissue space of the esophagus coincides with the organization of the intertwining of the lymphatic channels. The precise identification of the source of mucosal lymphatic capillaries is challenging and not definitively established. Some authors suggest the presence of precapillary spaces within the lamina mucosa, while others argue that true lymphatic capillaries may be absent in the middle and upper layers of the lamina mucosa.

Lymphatic capillaries within the esophagus first empty into lymphatic cisterns located within the submucosal layer. From there, they run along the muscular layer of the esophagus and distribute in a parallel fashion to the esophagus's long axis. The direction of lymphatic drainage

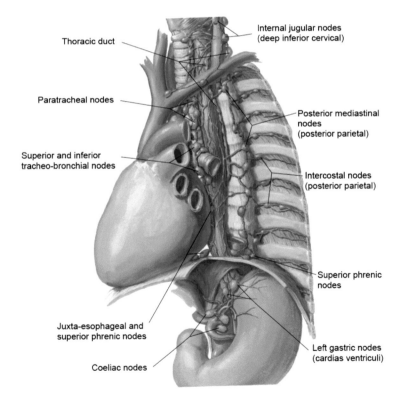

Figure 2.3 Lymphatic drainage of esophagus.

is determined by semilunar valves and collecting ducts. These collecting ducts ultimately open into peripheral lymph nodes after converging along several primary routes.

Lymphatic vessels from the proximal part of the esophagus drain into the cervical lymph nodes and subsequently enter the thoracic duct. Lymphatic vessels from the middle one-third of the esophagus drain into the posterior and superior lymph nodes in the mediastinum. Lastly, lymphatic vessels from the distal portion of the esophagus drain into the paracardial, left gastric, and celiac lymph nodes, following the path of the left gastric artery.

The presence of numerous lymphatic vessels make it possible for two directions of lymphatic drainage (ascending and descending), and in this way the spread of infection is explained.

2.2.5   Innervation of the Esophagus

The esophagus has a dual innervation, with sympathetic and parasympathetic nerve fibers. The vagal trunk consists of almost 80% afferent fibers, and the bodies of these cells project to the nucleus solitarius. In the muscle layer there are afferent fibers which are sensitive to mechanical stimuli. While through the afferent fibers, the innervation of the mucosa, the response to mechanical, thermal, chemical, and osmolar stimuli of the intraluminal space is realized. As previously mentioned, it is understood that these fibers transmit mechanical stimuli through mechanisms as pain, but they never directly transmit pain stimuli. Spinal afferent fibers follow a route starting from the dorsal ganglia where they have the cell body, ending in the nucleus gracilis and cuneatus. Impulse transmission is carried out through the mediation of the thalamus toward the cerebral insula and primary sensory areas.

The sensation of discomfort or pain is realized by the nerve endings in the muscular layer, functioning as a mechanoreceptor. Intraepithelial fibers are sensitive to pH stimuli and are activated upon exposure to acidic compounds. The vagus nerve holds the main place in the motor innervation of the esophagus, while the upper sphincter and the musculature of the proximal esophagus are innervated by efferent nerve fibers that end in the nucleus ambigus. In contrast, the innervation of the distal esophagus and the lower esophageal sphincter is provided by nerve fibers originating from the dorsal motor nucleus of the vagus nerve (see Figure 2.4).

The activity of secretory glands, the caliber of blood vessels, the activity of striated and smooth muscle fibers are controlled by the nerve fibers innervating the esophagus.

The innervation of the esophageal musculature and its secretory activity in terms of secretory glands is provided by parasympathetic nerve fibers of the dorsal nucleus of the vagus nerve as well as by the nucleus ambigus. While the regulation of sphincter contraction, relaxation of the esophageal musculature, stimulation of glandular secretion, esophageal peristalsis is achieved by the cervical and thoracic chain with projection from the first thoracic vertebra to the tenth.

Two types of nerve plexuses are distinguished in the wall of the esophagus: 1) Auerbach's plexus which is formed by the ganglions located between the circular and longitudinal muscle layers, and 2) Meissner's plexus, formed by the ganglions located in the submucosa layers.

Auerbach's plexus, whose nerve fibers are numerous in the esophageal smooth muscle, controls contractions of the external esophageal musculature and is primarily motor, while Meissner's plexus controls glandular secretion, peristalsis of submucosal muscle fibers, and is primarily sensorial. By running some imaging tests, it was noticed that the vagus nerve carries out the transmission of nerve impulses from the stimulation of

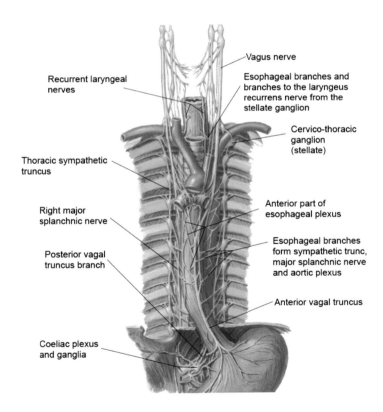

Figure 2.4 Innervation of esophagus.

nerve fibers in the esophagus and the latter are projected to the cerebral cortex through the thalamus and nerve centers. It is precisely the absence of these two plexuses in the distal part of the esophagus that leads to achalasia.

2.3   PHYSIOLOGY OF THE ESOPHAGUS

The esophagus is described as a muscular tube, whose main function is to transport the food bolus toward the stomach. The esophageal musculature undergoes a structural change in terms of the type of muscle composition. Specifically, the proximal part of the esophagus contains striated musculature, the distal part features smooth musculature, and the intermediate portion has a combination of both striated and smooth musculature.

2.3.1   The Process of Swallowing

This process starts when the food bolus passes from the oral cavity to the esophagus, passing through the upper esophageal sphincter, and is further executed by coordinating the relaxation of the upper sphincter with the contractions of the longitudinal and circular muscles.

2.3.2   Esophageal Peristalsis

The wave of esophageal peristalsis arises from the contraction of the circular esophageal musculature in a proximal to distal direction. Responsible for controlling this peristalsis is the medullary swallowing center with its afferent and efferent connections.

Auerbach's plexus, located between the muscular layers, has a major role in coordinating peristalsis in the distal esophagus.

As stated above, esophageal peristalsis is the result of sequential contractions of the circular muscles of the esophagus. There are three patterns of esophageal contractions, where we mention primary peristalsis, secondary peristalsis, and tertiary contractions.

Primary contractions represent the most common waveform resulting from the contraction of the circular musculature and progressing toward the distal esophagus; they are also initiated by several central mechanisms that follow the voluntary act of swallowing. The time for contraction waves to reach the distal part of the esophagus is about ten seconds, while the lower esophageal sphincter is relaxed throughout the time of primary peristalsis, except when peristalsis reaches this sphincter.

Secondary contractions begin as waves of circular muscle contraction that occur in response to esophageal distension. The primary role of secondary contractions is to clear the esophageal lumen of ingested material that has not been cleared by primary peristalsis. The resemblance to primary peristalsis is seen in the distal part of the esophagus where the waves take on a resemblance. Tertiary contractions were first discovered during barium X-ray studies and represent a wave of non-peristaltic contractions, while the physiological role of these contractions is unknown. The amplitude of the contractions is variable along the esophagus, where the distal and proximal parts predominate as those areas where the pressure is higher and the medial esophagus with an area of lower pressure. The existence of variable waves depending on the esophageal portion is best identified by high-resolution manometric studies. Speaking of a healthy individual, primary esophageal peristalsis is the initiation of waves after swallowing boluses of the same volume. When the swallows are 20 or 30 seconds apart, the amplitude and speed of the waves change, so while we are standing the amplitude of the waves is the lowest The speed of the waves are higher in the proximal esophagus than in the distal part. Both amplitude and speed decrease when we are consuming liquid food and increase when dry food is swallowed. Esophageal peristalsis has been shown to increase when large volumes of food boluses are swallowed, but this peristalsis has not been shown to be influenced by the age factor.

The muscles of the esophagus do not differ from each other only in the orientation of the muscle fibers but also in the response to the electrical stimulus. Based on this fact, the circular muscle, as long as the stimulus lasts, begins with a contraction and then is followed by a period of relaxation, the opposite happens with the longitudinal muscle where, for the duration of the stimulus, the muscle has a stable contraction. The time for the food bolus to go to the stomach is ten seconds, in this way, while swallowing begins, the longitudinal muscles contract and then provide a support for the contractions of the circular muscles, which, as stated above, makes a contraction and then relaxation of the entire esophagus.

Swallowing inhibition is the phenomenon that occurs when the swallows are between two to three seconds, and this inhibition is realized by the subsequent swallows which send inhibitory nerve signals. This inhibition is also called physiological inhibition due to the fact that the time in which it occurs is inappropriate and also the wave of peristalsis can damage the food bolus. Next is the latent period and the relaxation period, which clear the esophagus through a peristaltic contraction.

There are two components responsible for esophageal peristalsis, non-adrenergic and non-cholinergic mediators, where the most important role is played by nitric oxide and vasointestinal peptides.

Recent studies, in addition to peristaltic contractions, mostly support the fact that there is an esophageal compressive force. So, some researchers undertook an experiment, put a balloon in the esophagus, and the measured compressive force on the balloon was up to 200 gr. Thus, it was seen that the esophageal compressive force is greater in the distal esophagus and increases proportionally with the increase in the size and of the food bolus. It is the contractions of the circular and longitudinal muscles that create this compressive force, while at the moment the balloon is removed from the esophagus, this force is transformed into a peristaltic wave that advances distally.

BIBLIOGRAPHY

Rizvi S, Wehrle CJ, Law MA. StatPearls [Internet]. Treasure Island (FL): StatPearls Publishing; 2023 Jul 24. Anatomy, Thorax, Mediastinum Superior and Great Vessels.

Bains KNS, Kashyap S, Lappin SL. StatPearls [Internet]. Treasure Island (FL): StatPearls Publishing; 2023 Jul 24. Anatomy, Thorax, Diaphragm.

Mahabadi N, Goizueta AA, Bordoni B. StatPearls [Internet]. Treasure Island (FL): StatPearls Publishing; 2022 Oct 17. Anatomy, Thorax, Lung Pleura And Mediastinum.

Bardo DME, Biyyam DR, Patel MC, et al. Magnetic resonance imaging of the pediatric mediastinum. Pediatr Radiol. 2018 Aug;48(9):1209–22.

Ilahi M, St Lucia K, Ilahi TB. StatPearls [Internet]. Treasure Island (FL): StatPearls Publishing; 2023 Jul 24. Anatomy, Thorax, Thoracic Duct.

Fischer NJ, Morreau J, Sugunesegran R, et al. A reappraisal of pediatric thoracic surface anatomy. Clin Anat. 2017 Sep;30(6):788–94.

Bradley PJ. Symptoms and signs, staging and co-morbidity of hypopharyngeal cancer. Adv Otorhinolaryngol. 2019;83:15–26.

Sanghi V, Thota PN. Barrett's esophagus: Novel strategies for screening and surveillance. Ther Adv Chronic Dis. 2019;10:2040622319837851.

Gonzalez Ayerbe JI, Hauser B, Salvatore S, et al. Diagnosis and management of gastroesophageal reflux disease in infants and children: From guidelines to clinical practice. Pediatr Gastroenterol Hepatol Nutr. 2019 Mar;22(2):107–21.

Wolf DC. Dysphagia. In: Walker HK, Hall WD, Hurst JW, editors. Clinical methods: The history, physical, and laboratory examinations. 3rd ed. Boston: Butterworths; 1990.

Rishniw M, Rodriguez P, Que J, et al. Molecular aspects of esophageal development. Ann N Y Acad Sci. 2011 Sep;1232:309–15.

Que J. The initial establishment and epithelial morphogenesis of the esophagus: A new model of tracheal-esophageal separation and transition of simple columnar into stratified squamous epithelium in the developing esophagus. Wiley Interdiscip Rev Dev Biol. 2015 Jul–Aug;4(4):419–30.

Sivarao DV, Goyal RK. Functional anatomy and physiology of the upper esophageal sphincter. Am J Med. 2000 Mar 06;108(Suppl 4a):27S–37S.

Shaw SM, Martino R. The normal swallow: Muscular and neurophysiological control. Otolaryngol Clin North Am. 2013 Dec;46(6):937–56.

Mendell DA, Logemann JA. Temporal sequence of swallow events during the oropharyngeal swallow. J Speech Lang Hear Res. 2007 Oct;50(5):1256–71.

Goyal RK, Chaudhury A. Physiology of normal esophageal motility. J Clin Gastroenterol. 2008 May–Jun;42(5):610–19.

Brasseur JG, Nicosia MA, Pal A, et al. Function of longitudinal vs circular muscle fibers in esophageal peristalsis, deduced with mathematical modeling. World J Gastroenterol. 2007 Mar 07;13(9):1335–46.

Shiina T, Shima T, Wörl J, et al. The neural regulation of the mammalian esophageal motility and its implication for esophageal diseases. Pathophysiology. 2010 Apr;17(2):129–33.

Farré R, Sifrim D. Regulation of basal tone, relaxation and contraction of the lower oesophageal sphincter: Relevance to drug discovery for oesophageal disorders. Br J Pharmacol. 2008 Mar;153(5):858–69.

Kim HI, Hong SJ, Han JP, et al. Specific movement of esophagus during transient lower esophageal sphincter relaxation in gastroesophageal reflux disease. J Neurogastroenterol Motil. 2013 Jul;19(3):332–7.

Mittal RK. Motor function of the pharynx, esophagus, and its sphincters. San Rafael (CA): Morgan & Claypool Life Sciences; 2011.

Mittal RK. Regulation and dysregulation of esophageal peristalsis by the integrated function of circular and longitudinal muscle layers in health and disease. Am J Physiol Gastrointest Liver Physiol. 2016 Sep 01;311(3):G431–43.

Pickering M, Jones JF. The diaphragm: Two physiological muscles in one. J Anat. 2002 Oct;201(4):305–12.

Mittal RK. Esophageal function testing: Beyond manometry and impedance. Gastrointest Endosc Clin N Am. 2014 Oct;24(4):667–85.

Carlson DA, Pandolfino JE. High-resolution manometry in clinical practice. Gastroenterol Hepatol (N Y). 2015 Jun;11(6):374–84.

Roman S, Kahrilas PJ. Management of spastic disorders of the esophagus. Gastroenterol Clin North Am. 2013 Mar;42(1):27–43.

Ates F, Vaezi MF. The pathogenesis and management of achalasia: Current status and future directions. Gut Liver. 2015 Jul;9(4):449–63.

Ebert EC. Esophageal disease in scleroderma. J Clin Gastroenterol. 2006 Oct;40(9):769–75.

Martin RE, Letsos P, Taves DH, et al. Oropharyngeal dysphagia in esophageal cancer before and after transhiatal esophagectomy. Dysphagia. 2001 Winter;16(1):23–31.

Mamazza J, Schlachta CM, Poulin EC. Surgery for peptic strictures. Gastrointest Endosc Clin N Am. 1998 Apr;8(2):399–413.

DeVault KR. Lower esophageal (Schatzki's) ring: Pathogenesis, diagnosis and therapy. Dig Dis. 1996 Sep–Oct;14(5):323–9.

Law R, Katzka DA, Baron TH. Zenker's diverticulum. Clin Gastroenterol Hepatol. 2014 Nov;12(11):1773–82; quiz e111–12.

Chapter 3

Epidemiology of Esophageal Cancer

In relation to other cancerous diseases, esophageal tumors are the eighth most common type (3%), with a cumulative risk of 0.78% until the age of 74, in men 1.15% and in women 0.44%. A geographical distribution with higher incidence is observed in Eastern Asia and Eastern and Southern Africa, as well as in countries with a high development index (HDI). Esophageal cancer has a five-year survival rate of around 20%, but this rate varies widely, ranging from 5% to 50%. This variability can be attributed to factors such as late-stage diagnosis and the high aggressiveness of the cancer.

Barrett's esophagus is the most significant precancerous condition associated with esophageal cancer. Individuals with Barrett's esophagus have a risk up to 100 times higher than the general population of developing esophageal cancer. These patients require regular monitoring to detect tumors at an early, treatable stage. However, it's important to note that not all individuals with Barrett's esophagus will develop esophageal cancer. Some population-based cohort studies have reported an incidence of 0.1% to 0.2% of esophageal adenocarcinoma in patients with Barrett's esophagus.

In many countries, including the United States, esophageal and gastro-esophageal junction cancers are relatively rare. Regarding the location of esophageal cancer, the incidence of cancer in the distal one-third of the esophagus is roughly equal to that in the proximal two-thirds. Globally, squamous cell carcinoma is the most common histological type of esophageal cancer. The incidence of squamous cell carcinoma increases with age and typically peaks in the seventh decade of life. In terms of race and gender, squamous cell carcinoma is three times more common in populations of African descent, while adenocarcinomas are more prevalent in Caucasian men. The risk of various types of esophageal cancer generally increases with age, with a median age of diagnosis around 67 years. In African populations the incidence is about twice as high as in Caucasian populations. Squamous cell carcinoma is diagnosed mostly in

DOI: 10.1201/9781003497547-3

black people and white women, while adenocarcinoma is more common in white men.

This disease is a major global threat. It is four times more frequent in men and with higher mortality than in women. Geographically, esophageal cancer is up to 30 times more common in China than in the United States. It is noted that a link between environment, diet, and esophageal cancer exists, starting from the drastic difference in incidence in different parts of the globe. There appears to be a "hot" zone stretching from northeast China to the Middle East. The risk factors seem to be those that have a direct impact on the esophagus and less of those that have a systemic impact. Initially, alcohol consumption and poverty, which may cause local damage and systemic nutrient insufficiency, cannot fully explain the reason for this incidence. The presence of other carcinogenic factors may explain this situation. It is thought that the best method to reduce the incidence of this disease is to reduce the development of esophagitis caused by nutrition and food culture.

3.1   RISK FACTORS

The mechanisms of carcinogenesis of esophageal tumors are not fully understood, and over the years the type of adenocarcinoma is appearing more and more.

Smoking and alcohol consumption are among the main factors in the development of squamous cell carcinoma of the esophagus. Recently, obesity is emerging as a strong risk factor for increasing the incidence of adenocarcinoma. Numerous studies indicate a three-fold risk for overweight individuals.

The use of red meat in the diet, smoking, and consumption of "shisha" smoke, chewing tobacco products, opiates, poor oral hygiene, low socioeconomic status, low consumption of fresh fruits and vegetables, as well as hot drinks are behaviors associated with increased risk for squamous cell carcinoma. As for esophageal adenocarcinoma, Barrett's disease is clearly recognized as a risk factor.

3.1.1   Smoking

Individuals who regularly consume tobacco products have a high risk of developing both adenocarcinoma and squamous cell carcinoma of the esophagus. Studies show that ingesting tobacco smoke residues exposes the esophageal mucosa to carcinogenic substances, such as nitrosamines. The duration and number of cigarettes consumed have a direct impact on increasing the risk of esophageal cancer.

3.1.2   Inflammation and Irritation of the Mucous Membrane

The presence of esophageal irritant factors such as alcohol consumption, food retention in the esophagus (release of chemical irritants from bacterial decomposition), frequent consumption of hot drinks and their combination with tobacco consumption seem to cause a significant increase in the development of carcinoma squamous cells of the esophagus. Factors such as esophageal achalasia, H. pylori, and HPV infections may also be involved.

Individuals who have a history of ingesting corrosive substances such as acids, bases, pesticides, and detergents also have an approximately 5% risk of developing esophageal cancer in the next five years.

3.1.3   Obesity

Socio-economic status is a factor which is clearly related to the development of squamous cell carcinoma. Western developed countries which in recent decades are showing an increased prevalence of obese people are showing an increasing incidence of adenocarcinoma of the esophagus. This is thought to be related to gastroesophageal reflux (GERD) resulting from increased intra-abdominal pressure. On the other hand, the increase of adipose tissue also predisposes to the release of tumor development factors such as cytokines and adipokines. The abundant presence of fats in adipocytes forms a suitable environment for uncontrolled tumor growth.

3.1.4   Genetics

The genetic factors that influence the development of adenocarcinoma of the esophagus are not clearly known, however, genomic studies have been carried out to understand more about the alleles that predispose to this disease. Howel-Evans, a rare autosomal dominant syndrome characterized by palmar and plantar hyperkeratosis and esophageal papillomatosis appears to have a high risk of developing squamous cell carcinoma.

Paterson-Kelly syndrome which manifests with dysphagia, odynophagia, angular cheilitis, iron deficiency anemia, and the development of web-like membranes predisposes to the occurrence of esophageal cancer.

3.1.5   Demography

It was discussed previously that the incidence of esophageal cancer increases with increasing age and peaks in the seventh decade of life, the higher predisposition of men over women as well as the black population.

BIBLIOGRAPHY

Sung H, Ferlay J, Siegel RL, et al. Global cancer statistics 2020: GLOBOCAN estimates of incidence and mortality worldwide for 36 cancers in 185 countries. CA Cancer J Clin. 2021;71:209–49. doi: 10.3322/caac.21660.

Siegel RL, Miller KD, Fuchs HE, et al. Cancer statistics, 2021. CA Cancer J Clin. 2021;71:7–33. doi: 10.3322/caac.21654.

Merkow RP, Bilimoria KY, Keswani RN, et al. Treatment trends, risk of lymph node metastasis, and outcomes for localized esophageal cancer. J Natl Cancer Inst. 2014;106:dju133. doi: 10.1093/jnci/dju133.

Cao W, Chen HD, Yu YW, et al. Changing profiles of cancer burden worldwide and in China: A secondary analysis of the global cancer statistics 2020. Chin Med J (Engl). 2021;134:783–91. doi: 10.1097/CM9.0000000000001474.

Zheng RS, Sun KX, Zhang SW, et al. Report of cancer epidemiology in China, 2015. Zhonghua Zhong Liu Za Zhi. 2019;41:19–28. doi: 10.3760/cma.j.issn.0253-3766.2019.01.005.

Thrumurthy SG, Chaudry MA, Thrumurthy SSD, et al. Oesophageal cancer: Risks, prevention, and diagnosis. BMJ. 2019;366:l4373. doi: 10.1136/bmj.l4373.

Fitzgerald RC, di Pietro M, Ragunath K, et al. British Society of Gastroenterology guidelines on the diagnosis and management of Barrett's oesophagus. Gut. 2014;63:7–42. doi: 10.1136/gutjnl-2013-305372.

American Gastroenterological Association, Spechler SJ, Sharma P, et al. American Gastroenterological Association medical position statement on the management of Barrett's esophagus. Gastroenterol. 2011;140:1084–91. doi: 10.1053/j.gastro.2011.01.030.

Asge Standards of Practice Committee, Qumseya B, Sultan S, et al. ASGE guideline on screening and surveillance of Barrett's esophagus. Gastrointest Endosc. 2019;90:335–59.e2. doi: 10.1016/j.gie.2019.05.012.

Shaheen NJ, Falk GW, Iyer PG, et al. ACG clinical guideline: Diagnosis and management of Barrett's esophagus. Am J Gastroenterol. 2016;111:30–50;quiz 51. doi: 10.1038/ajg.2015.322.

National Clinical Research Center for Digestive Diseases, Chinese Digestive Endoscopy Society, Chinese Digestive Doctor Association. The Chinese consensus for screening, diagnosis and management of Barrett's esophagus and early adenocarcinoma (2017, Wanning). Zhonghua Nei Ke Za Zhi. 2017;56:701–11. doi: 10.3760/cma.j.issn.0578-1426.2017.09.020.

National Digestive Endoscopy Quality Control Center, National Clinical Research Center for Digestive Diseases (Shanghai), National Early Gastrointestinal-Cancer Prevention & Treatment Center Alliance (GECA), et al. China experts consensus on screening of early esophageal cancer and pre-cancerous lesion screening (2019, Xinxiang). Zhonghua Xiao Hua Nei Jing Za Zhi. 2019;36:793–801. doi: 10.3760/cma.j.issn.1007-5232.2019.11.001.

Chinese Society of Digestive Endoscopy, Chinese Society of Gastroenterology. Chinese consensus: Screening, diagnosis and treatment of early esophageal squamous cell carcinoma and precancerous lesions (2015, Beijing).

Zhonghua Nei Ke Za Zhi. 2016;55:73–85. doi: 10.3760/cma.j.issn.0578-1426.2016.01.016.

Chinese Society of Digestive Endoscopy, Cancer Endoscopy Professional Committee of China Anti-Cancer Association. Chinese expert consensus on screening and endoscopic management of early esophageal cancer (Beijing, 2014). Zhonghua Shi Yong Nei Ke Za Zhi. 2015;35:320–37. doi: 10.7504/nk2015030402.

Bray F, Ferlay J, Soerjomataram I, et al. Global cancer statistics 2018: GLOBOCAN estimates of incidence and mortality worldwide for 36 cancers in 185 countries. CA Cancer J Clin. 2018;68:394–424. doi: 10.3322/caac.21492.

GBD 2019 Diseases and Injuries Collaborators. Global burden of 369 diseases and injuries in 204 countries and territories, 1990–2019: A systematic analysis for the Global Burden of Disease Study 2019. Lancet. 2020;396:1204–22. doi: 10.1016/S0140-6736(20)30925-9.

Chen F, Wang YQ. Disease burden and trends of esophageal cancer in China during 1990–2019. Zhongguo Zhong Liu. 2021;30:401–7. doi: 10.11735/j.issn.1004-0242.2021.06.A001.

Liang H, Fan JH, Qiao YL. Epidemiology, etiology, and prevention of esophageal squamous cell carcinoma in China. Cancer Bio Med. 2017;14:33–41. doi: 10.20892/j.issn.2095-3941.2016.0093.

Lu CL, Lang HC, Luo JC, et al. Increasing trend of the incidence of esophageal squamous cell carcinoma, but not adenocarcinoma, in Taiwan. Cancer Causes Control. 2010;21:269–74. doi: 10.1007/s10552-009-9458-0.

Schneider JL, Corley DA. A review of the epidemiology of Barrett's oesophagus and oesophageal adenocarcinoma. Best Pract Res Clin Gastroenterol. 2015;29:29–39. doi: 10.1016/j.bpg.2014.11.008.

Thrift AP. The epidemic of oesophageal carcinoma: Where are we now? Cancer Epidemiol. 2016;41:88–95.

Tran GD, Sun XD, Abnet CC, et al. Prospective study of risk factors for esophageal and gastric cancers in the Linxian general population trial cohort in China. Int J Cancer. 2005;113:456–63. doi: 10.1002/ijc.20616.

He Z, Zhao Y, Guo C, et al. Prevalence and risk factors for esophageal squamous cell cancer and precursor lesions in Anyang, China: A population-based endoscopic survey. Br J Cancer. 2010;103:1085–8. doi: 10.1038/sj.bjc.6605843.

Lin Y, Totsuka Y, Shan B, et al. Esophageal cancer in high-risk areas of China: Research progress and challenges. Ann Epidemiol. 2017;27:215–21. doi: 10.1016/j.annepidem.2016.11.004.

Abnet CC, Arnold M, Wei WQ. Epidemiology of esophageal squamous cell carcinoma. Gastroenterol. 2018;154:360–73. doi: 10.1053/j.gastro.2017.08.023.

Lin Y, Totsuka Y, He Y, et al. Epidemiology of esophageal cancer in Japan and China. J Epidemiol. 2013;23:233–42. doi: 10.2188/jea.je20120162.

Zhou MG, Wang XF, Hu JP, et al. Geographical distribution of cancer mortality in China, 2004–2005. Zhonghua Yu Fang Yi Xue Za Zhi. 2010;44:303–8. doi: 10.3760/cma.j.issn.0253-9624.2010.04.006.

Zeng HM, Zheng RS, Zhang SW, et al. Analysis and prediction of esophageal cancer incidence trend in China. Zhonghua Yu Fang Yi Xue Za Zhi. 2012;46:593–7. doi: 10.3760/cma.j.issn.0253-9624.2012.07.004.

American Cancer Society. Cancer statistics 2021 report. J Nucl Med 2021;62:12N.

Pohl H, Sirovich B, Welch HG. Esophageal adenocarcinoma incidence: Are we reaching the peak? Cancer Epidemiol Biomarkers Prev. 2010;19:1468–70.

Chapter 4

Classification of Esophageal Cancer

4.1 BENIGN TUMORS OF THE ESOPHAGUS

Compared to esophageal carcinoma, benign tumors are uncommon. They are observed in about 5% of biopsies of resected tumor masses. Clinically, benign tumors may be asymptomatic, but require constant surveillance due to their size or even the ambiguity of histological nature.

Due to a mild clinic, these tumors are diagnosed incidentally during endoscopic or imaging procedures that are performed for other reasons. In cases where the tumor becomes clinically significant, it may begin with signs of dysphagia, regurgitation, ulceration, and hemorrhage. Another important symptom is pain, mainly retrosternal or epigastric, accompanied by heartburn, as well as obstructive signs. This may coincide with a tumor that exceeds 5 cm in diameter.

Among the most valuable diagnostic modalities we can mention:

- Radiography with oral barium contrast, as an initial method for evaluating a patient with swallowing difficulties.
- CT scanner to evaluate the extent of the tumor, the relationships with the anatomical structures, but also the exclusion of any mediastinal mass which mimics the clinical features of an esophageal tumor.
- Endoscopy and echoendoscopy are very important for the clear visualization of the endoluminal view, taking the biopsy as well as the characteristics of the layers of the esophagus wall.

The most common benign tumors of the esophagus can be classified according to localization in intramural, intraluminal, and extraesophageal layers, namely:

- *Intramural*
  - Leiomyoma.
  - Gastrointestinal stromal tumor (GIST) or Schwannoma.

DOI: 10.1201/9781003497547-4

- *Intraluminal*
  - Inflammatory epithelial polyps.
  - Adenomatous epithelial polyps.
  - Fibrovascular polyps.
  - Hemangioma.
  - Papilloma.
  - Granular cell tumors.
- *Extraesophageal*
  - Congenital esophageal cysts and duplications.

4.2 MALIGNANT ESOPHAGEAL TUMORS

As we mentioned extensively in the chapters above, the main malignant tumors of the esophagus are adenocarcinoma of the esophagus and squamous cell carcinoma.

Over the years, different protocols have been applied for the classification of esophageal tumors in order to accurately stage the disease to enable the maximum therapeutic benefit to the patient. This is based on imaging, endoscopic, histopathological data, and prognostic progress pre- and post-intervention, and radio-chemotherapy. Currently the most recent and widely accepted proposal for esophageal cancer is the eighth version of the American Joint Committee on Cancer (AJCC).

4.2.1 Anatomical Features, Tumor Localization

Anatomically, the esophagus is divided into three portions, cervical, thoracic, and abdominal, but in relation to the distance from the incisor teeth it can be divided into the upper, middle, and lower one-third. However, the relationship of the tumor with the surrounding structures is of greater importance than its longitudinal positioning.

4.2.1.1 Cervical Esophagus

The cervical esophagus lies in the neck region, bordered from above by the hypopharynx and below by the thoracic hiatus, at the level of the jugular incisor of the sternum. It is limited to the carotid sheath, vertebrae, and trachea. In endoscopic measurements, depending on the anatomical structure of the patient, the lower border of the cervical esophagus is 15–20 cm from the incisor teeth. In the CT scan, this border is defined by the jugular incision of the sternum.

4.2.1.2 Upper Thoracic Esophagus

It is bounded by the thoracic hiatus superiorly and the azygos vein inferiorly. In the anterior and lateral parts, there are relations with the trachea, the vessels of the aortic arch, and the great veins, while posteriorly it is limited by the vertebrae. In endoscopic measurements, this length corresponds to a distance of 20–25 cm from the incisors.

4.2.1.3 Middle Thoracic Esophagus

Located between the superior boundary marked by the azygos vein and the inferior boundary formed by the inferior pulmonary veins. It has anatomical relationships with the vertebrae, the thoracic aorta, and the pulmonary hilus. When examined endoscopically, it is typically found at a distance of 25–30 cm from the incisor teeth.

On the other hand, the lower thoracic esophagus and the gastroesophageal junction are situated between the superior boundary represented by the inferior pulmonary veins and the inferior boundary formed by the stomach. This portion of the esophagus has anatomical connections with the vertebrae, the descending thoracic aorta, and the pericardium, ultimately passing through the diaphragmatic hiatus. In terms of endoscopic measurements, this region corresponds to a distance of approximately 30–40 cm from the incisors.

Some notions for the classification of malignant esophageal tumors are found in Table 4.1.

Table 4.1 TNM Classification

T class	Description and criteria
Tx	Tumor cannot be evaluated
T0	No evidence of tumor
Tis	Tumor in situ, cancerous cells do not pass the basal membrane
T1a	Tumor passes into lamina propria or muscularis mucosae
T1b	Tumor passes into submucosa
T2	Tumor invades muscularis propria layer
T3	Tumor invades adventitia layer
T4a	Tumor involves nearby structures such as pleura, pericardium, azygos vein, diaphragm, or peritoneum
T4b	Tumor involves further structures such as aorta, vertebral bodies, and airways
N class	Description and criteria
Nx	Locoregional lymph nodes cannot be evaluated
N0	No lymphonodal involvement
N1	One to two affected regional lymph nodes
N2	Three to six affected regional lymph nodes
N3	Seven or more affected regional lymph nodes
M class	Description and criteria
Mx	Distant metastases cannot be evaluated
M0	No distant metastases
M1	Distant metastases present

Table 4.2 Differentiation Grade for Esophageal Adenocarcinoma

G class	Description and criteria
G I	A well-differentiated tumor, where over 95% is composed of glandular structures
G II	A moderately differentiated tumor, where 50% up to 95% is composed of glandular structures (example Figure 4.1)
G III	A poorly differentiated tumor which has no glandular structures, or less than 50% is composed of glandular structures

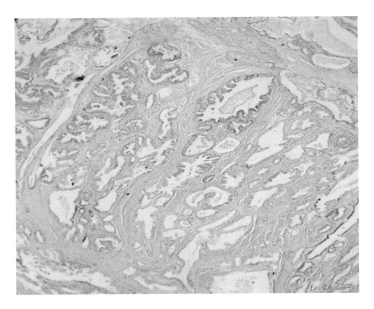

Figure 4.1 Moderately differentiated esophageal adenocarcinoma (GII)—Pathology Department QSUT.

Table 4.3 Differentiation Grade for Squamous Cell Esophageal Cancer

G class	Description and criteria
G I	A well-differentiated tumor, with low mitosis index. Cells are organized in layers, with pearl keratinization and few elements of basal-type non keratinizing cells.
G II	A moderately differentiated tumor, with variable histologic presentation from lesions with initial keratinization to lesions with poor keratinization, without pearl formation (example Figure 4.2)
G III	A poorly differentiated tumor which has a nest-like structure with basal cells and often central necrosis. These structures are formed by layers of cancerous cells organized in tiles, with spots of keratinizing cells.

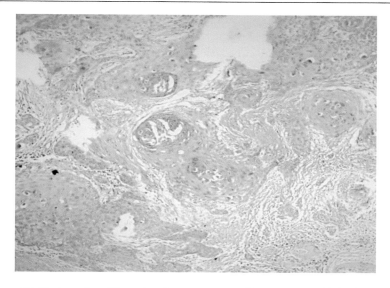

Figure 4.2 Moderately differentiated squamous cell carcinoma (GII)—Pathology Department QSUT.

4.3 ESOPHAGEAL CANCER STAGING

Groupings for the classification of esophageal cancer are based on the systematic arrangement according to the extent of the primary tumor (T), and then also according to lymphatic metastasis (N) and other organ spread (M). These data, together with a prognostic analysis of the survival of esophageal cancer cases on a global scale, have made it possible to stage this pathology. This staging is subject to continuous change in light of new data and improved statistical analysis.

Because of the peculiarities of esophageal cancer and its lymphatic anatomy, it is possible for superficial, low T-grade tumors to have lymphnodal involvement. This would make the prognosis of the cancer comparable to a more advanced Stage T tumor but with Grade N0 (see Table 4.4). Also, the prognosis of esophageal cancer depends on the degree of differentiation, the type of tumor and the anatomical location.

Esophageal cancer staging aims to determine which patient may benefit from surgical intervention. Thus, Stages I and II are considered potentially resectable. In some cases of Stage III, when there is no infiltration of the trachea or large vessels, the tumor can be considered resectable, but often the patients are not suitable candidates for intervention. Tumors that have infiltrated the surrounding structures or spread to distant lymph nodes are considered unresectable and surgical intervention is not indicated.

Table 4.4 Pathologic Stadification for Squamous Cell Carcinoma

T class	N class	M class	Grade	Localization	Stage
Tis	N0	M0	No evaluation	Any localization	0
T1a	N0	M0	G I	Any localization	IA
T1a	N0	M0	G II–III	Any localization	IB
T1a	N0	M0	G X	Any localization	IA
T1b	N0	M0	G I–III	Any localization	IB
T1b	N0	M0	G X	Any localization	IB
T2	N0	M0	G I	Any localization	IB
T2	N0	M0	G II–III	Any localization	IIA
T2	N0	M0	G X	Any localization	IIA
T3	N0	M0	Any G	Lower portion	IIA
T3	N0	M0	G I	Upper/Middle	IIA
T3	N0	M0	G II–III	Upper/Middle	IIB
T3	N0	M0	G X	Any localization	IIB
T3	N0	M0	Any G	Localization X	IIB
T1	N1	M0	Any G	Any localization	IIB
T1	N2	M0	Any G	Any localization	IIIA
T2	N1	M0	Any G	Any localization	IIIA
T2	N2	M0	Any G	Any localization	IIIB
T3	N1–N2	M0	Any G	Any localization	IIIB
T4a	N0–N1	M0	Any G	Any localization	IIIB
T4a	N2	M0	Any G	Any localization	IVA
T4b	N0–N2	M0	Any G	Any localization	IVA
Any T	N3	M0	Any G	Any localization	IVA
Any T	Any N	M1	Any G	Any localization	IVB

Table 4.5 Description of Squamous Cell Carcinoma Stages

Stage	Description
0	The tumor is located in the epithelial lining of the esophagus and did not penetrate deeper layers. Can have any location in the esophagus. No differentiation grades applicable
IA	Tumor is invading lamina propria or muscularis mucosae and has no lymph node involvement or metastases. It is of Grade I or unknown grade of differentiation
IB	Tumor is invading lamina propria, muscularis mucosae, submucosa, or muscularis propria, but has no affected lymph nodes or metastases. Can be of any grade
IIA	Tumor has invaded muscularis propria but has no affected lymph nodes or distant organs. Has a Grade II–III or unknown grade [or] Tumor has invaded the outer layer of esophagus, adventitia, but has no lymph nodes or metastases. Can be of any grade and localized in the lower third portion or Grade I and localized in the upper and middle one-third

Stage	Description
IIB	Tumor has passed into adventitia and has no lymph nodes or metastases. Has a Grade I–II with localization in upper and middle esophagus; can be of unknown grade and localization in any portion of esophagus; or any grade and unknown localization [or] Tumor has invaded lamina propria, muscularis mucosae, or the submucosa. One to two lymph nodes are affected. Can have any grade and any localization
IIIA	Tumor has invaded lamina propria, muscularis mucosae, submucosa, or muscularis propria. Has no more than six affected lymph nodes and no metastases. Can be of any grade or localization
IIIB	Tumor may have invaded: 1) muscularis propria, but no more than six lymph nodes; 2) adventitia, but no more than six lymph nodes; 3) has infiltrated pleura, pericardium, or diaphragm, but has no more than two lymph nodes Has no metastases. Can be of any grade and localization
IVA	Tumor has involved: 1) the pleura, pericardium, or diaphragm, but no more than six affected lymph nodes; 2) trachea, aorta, vertebral bodies, and other important structures, but no more than six lymph nodes; 3) may have affected any esophageal layer and has seven or more lymph nodes Can be of any grade and localization in the esophagus
IVB	Tumor has involved distant lymph nodes or organs such as lungs and liver. Can be of any grade and can be localized anywhere in esophagus

Table 4.6 Pathologic Classification for Adenocarcinoma

T class	N class	M class	Grade	Stage
Tis	N0	M0	No evaluation	0
T1a	N0	M0	G I	IA
T1a	N0	M0	G X	IA
T1a	N0	M0	G II	IB
T1b	N0	M0	G I–II	IB
T1b	N0	M0	G X	IB
T1	N0	M0	G III	IC
T2	N0	M0	G I-II	IC
T2	N0	M0	G III	IIA
T2	N0	M0	G X	IIA
T1	N1	M0	Any G	IIB
T3	N0	M0	Any G	IIB
T1	N2	M0	Any G	IIIA
T2	N1	M0	Any G	IIIA
T2	N2	M0	Any G	IIIB
T3	N1–N2	M0	Any G	IIIB
T4a	N0–N1	M0	Any G	IIIB
T4a	N2	M0	Any G	IVA
T4b	N0–N2	M0	Any G	IVA
Any T	N3	M0	Any G	IVA
Any T	Any N	M1	Any G	IVB

Table 4.7 Stage Description for Esophageal Adenocarcinoma

Stage	Definition
0	Tumor is located in the epithelial lining of the esophagus and has not passed into other layers. Can be located anywhere in the esophageal length. No differentiation grades are applicable
IA	Tumor is developing in lamina propria or muscularis mucosae, without lymph node involvement or metastases. It is of Grade I or unknown differentiation grade
IB	Tumor is developing in lamina propria, muscularis mucosae, or submucosa, but has no lymph nodes or metastases. May be of Grade I–II or of unknown differentiation grade
IC	Tumor is evolving in lamina propria, muscularis mucosae, submucosa, or muscularis propria. It has no affected lymph nodes. Can be of Grade I–III
IIA	Tumor has infiltrated muscularis propria. It has no lymph node involvement. May be of Grade III or of unknown grade
IIB	Tumor has invaded lamina propria, muscularis mucosae, or submucosa. It has one to two affected regional nodes. It is of any grade and has no metastases [or] Tumor has invaded adventitia. It is of any grade and has no lymph node involvement
IIIA	Tumor has infiltrated lamina propria, muscularis mucosae, submucosa, and muscularis propria. It has no more than six affected lymph nodes. Has no metastases and may be of any grade of differentiation
IIIB	Tumor may have invaded: 1) muscularis propria, but no more than six affected lymph nodes; 2) adventitia, but no more than six affected lymph nodes; 3) pleura, pericardium, or diaphragm, but no more than two affected lymph nodes Has no metastatic spread and can be of any differentiation grade
IVA	Tumor has invaded: 1) pleura, pericardium, or diaphragm with no more than six affected lymph nodes; 2) trachea, aorta, vertebral column, or other major structures, but no more than six affected lymph nodes; 3) any esophageal layer, but has seven or more affected regional lymph nodes Any differentiation grade
IVB	Tumor has affected distant lymph nodes or organs such as the lungs or the liver. Can be of any differentiation grade

BIBLIOGRAPHY

Rice TW, Kelsen DP, Blackstone EH, et al. Esophagus and esophagogastric junction. In: Amin MB, Edge SB, Greene FL, et al., editors. AJCC cancer staging manual. 8th ed. New York: Springer; 2017. p. 185–202.

Rice TW, Chen LQ, Hofstetter WL, et al. Worldwide esophageal cancer collaboration: Pathologic staging data. Dis Esophagus. 2016;29:724–33. doi: 10.1111/dote.12520.

Rice TW, Apperson-Hansen C, DiPaola LM, et al. World wide esophageal cancer collaboration: Clinical staging data. Dis Esophagus. 2016;29:707–14. doi: 10.1111/dote.12493.

Rice TW, Lerut TE, Orringer MB, et al. Worldwide esophageal cancer collaboration: Neoadjuvant pathologic staging data. Dis Esophagus. 2016;29:715–23. doi: 10.1111/dote.12513.

Rice TW, Ishwaran H, Hofstetter WL, et al. Recommendations for pathologic staging (pTNM) of cancer of the esophagus and esophagogastric junction for the 8th edition AJCC/UICC staging manuals. Dis Esophagus. 2016;29:897–905.

Rice TW, Ishwaran H, Blackstone EH, et al. Recommendations for clinical staging (cTNM) of cancer of the esophagus and esophagogastric junction for the 8th edition AJCC/UICC staging manuals. Dis Esophagus. 2016;29:913–19.

Rice TW, Ishwaran H, Kelsen DP, et al. Recommendations for neoadjuvant pathologic staging (ypTNM) of cancer of the esophagus and esophagogastric junction for the 8th edition AJCC/UICC staging manuals. Dis Esophagus. 2016;29:906–12.

Cancer Genome Atlas Research Network. Comprehensive molecular characterization of gastric adenocarcinoma. Nature. 2014;513:202–9. doi: 10.1038/nature13480.

Hayakawa Y, Sethi N, Sepulveda AR, et al. Oesophageal adenocarcinoma and gastric cancer: Should we mind the gap? Nat Rev Cancer. 2016;16:305–18. doi: 10.1038/nrc.2016.24.

Montgomery E, Field JK, Boffetta P. Squamous cell carcinoma of the oesophagus. In: Bosman FT, Carneiro F, Hruban RH, et al., editors. WHO classification of tumours of the digestive system. 4th ed. Lyon: International Agency for Research on Cancer; 2010. p. 18–24.

Flejou JF, Odze RD, Montgomery E, et al. Adenocarcinoma of the oesophagus. In: Bosman FT, Carneiro F, Hruban RH, et al., editors. WHO classification of tumours of the digestive system. 4th ed. Lyon: International Agency for Research on Cancer; 2010. p. 25–31.

Chirieac LR, Swisher SG, Correa AM, et al. Signet-ring cell or mucinous histology after preoperative chemoradiation and survival in patients with esophageal or esophagogastric junction adenocarcinoma. Clin Cancer Res. 2005;11:2229–36. doi: 10.1158/1078-0432.CCR-04-1840.

Kelly S, Harris KM, Berry E, et al. A systematic review of the staging performance of endoscopic ultrasound in gastro-oesophageal carcinoma. Gut. 2001;49:534–9. doi: 10.1136/gut.49.4.534.

Rice TW, Ishwaran H, Hofstetter WL, et al. Esophageal cancer: Associations with (pN+) lymph node metastases. Ann Surg. 2017;265:122–9. doi: 10.1097/SLA.0000000000001594.

Barbour AP, Rizk NP, Gerdes H, et al. Endoscopic ultrasound predicts outcomes for patients with adenocarcinoma of the gastroesophageal junction. J Am Coll Surg. 2007;205:593–601. doi: 10.1016/j.jamcollsurg.2007.05.010.

Blackshaw G, Lewis WG, Hopper AN, et al. Prospective comparison of endosonography, computed tomography, and histopathological stage of junctional oesophagogastric cancer. Clin Radiol. 2008;63:1092–8. doi: 10.1016/j.crad.2008.04.006.

Murata Y, Napoleon B, Odegaard S. High-frequency endoscopic ultrasonography in the evaluation of superficial esophageal cancer. Endoscopy. 2003;35:429–35; discussion 436. doi: 10.1055/s-2003-38774.

Puli SR, Reddy JB, Bechtold ML, et al. Staging accuracy of esophageal cancer by endoscopic ultrasound: A meta-analysis and systematic review. World J Gastroenterol. 2008;14:1479–90. doi: 10.3748/wjg.14.1479.

Rice TW, Mason DP, Murthy SC, et al. T2N0M0 esophageal cancer. J Thorac Cardiovasc Surg. 2007;133:317–24. doi: 10.1016/j.jtcvs.2006.09.023.

Hardacker TJ, Ceppa D, Okereke I, et al. Treatment of clinical T2N0M0 esophageal cancer. Ann Surg Oncol. 2014;21:3739–43. doi: 10.1245/s10434-014-3929-6.

Thota PN, Sada A, Sanaka MR, et al. Correlation between endoscopic forceps biopsies and endoscopic mucosal resection with endoscopic ultrasound in patients with Barrett's esophagus with high-grade dysplasia and early cancer. Surg Endosc. 2017;31:1336–41. doi: 10.1007/s00464-016-5117-1.

Pimentel-Nunes P, Dinis-Ribeiro M, Ponchon T, et al. Endoscopic submucosal dissection: European Society of Gastrointestinal Endoscopy (ESGE) guideline. Endoscopy. 2015;47:829–54. doi: 10.1055/s-0034-1392882.

Yang D, Coman RM, Kahaleh M, et al. Endoscopic submucosal dissection for Barrett's early neoplasia: A multicenter study in the United States. Gastrointest Endosc. 2016. [Epub ahead of print]. doi: 10.1016/j.gie.2016.09.023.

Gress DM, Edge SB, Greene FL, et al. Principles of cancer staging. In: Amin MB, Edge SB, Greene FL, et al., editors. AJCC cancer staging manual. 8th ed. New York: Springer; 2017. p. 3–30.

Kutup A, Link BC, Schurr PG, et al. Quality control of endoscopic ultrasound in preoperative staging of esophageal cancer. Endoscopy. 2007;39:715–19. doi: 10.1055/s-2007-966655.

van Overhagen H, Becker CD. Diagnosis and staging of carcinoma of the esophagus and gastroesophageal junction, and detection of postoperative recurrence, by computed tomography. In: Meyers M, editor. Neoplasms of the digestive tract: Imaging, staging and management. Philadelphia: Lippincott-Raven; 1998. p. 31–48.

Doi N, Aoyama N, Tokunaga M, et al. Possibility of pre-operative diagnosis of lymph node metastasis based on morphology. Hepatogastroenterology. 1999;46:977–80.

van Vliet EP, Heijenbrok-Kal MH, Hunink MG, et al. Staging investigations for oesophageal cancer: A meta-analysis. Br J Cancer. 2008;98:547–57. doi: 10.1038/sj.bjc.6604200.

Flanagan FL, Dehdashti F, Siegel BA, et al. Staging of esophageal cancer with 18F-fluorodeoxyglucose positron emission tomography. AJR Am J Roentgenol. 1997;168:417–24. doi: 10.2214/ajr.168.2.9016218.

Kato H, Kuwano H, Nakajima M, et al. Comparison between positron emission tomography and computed tomography in the use of the assessment of esophageal carcinoma. Cancer 2002;94:921–8. doi: 10.1002/cncr.10330.

Flamen P, Lerut A, Van Cutsem E, et al. Utility of positron emission tomography for the staging of patients with potentially operable esophageal carcinoma. J Clin Oncol. 2000;18:3202–10. doi: 10.1200/JCO.2000.18.18.3202.

Roedl JB, Blake MA, Holalkere NS, et al. Lymph node staging in esophageal adenocarcinoma with PET-CT based on a visual analysis and based on metabolic parameters. Abdom Imaging. 2009;34:610–17. doi: 10.1007/s00261-008-9447-x.

Choi J, Kim SG, Kim JS, et al. Comparison of endoscopic ultrasonography (EUS), positron emission tomography (PET), and computed tomography (CT) in the preoperative locoregional staging of resectable esophageal cancer. Surg Endosc. 2010;24:1380–6. doi: 10.1007/s00464-009-0783-x.

Wiersema MJ, Vilmann P, Giovannini M, et al. Endosonography-guided fine-needle aspiration biopsy: Diagnostic accuracy and complication assessment. Gastroenterol. 1997;112:1087–95. doi: 10.1016/S0016-5085(97)70164-1.

Bergman JJ. The endoscopic diagnosis and staging of oesophageal adenocarcinoma. Best Pract Res Clin Gastroenterol. 2006;20:843–66. doi: 10.1016/j.bpg.2006.04.010.

Giovannini M, Seitz JF, Monges G, et al. Fine-needle aspiration cytology guided by endoscopic ultrasonography: Results in 141 patients. Endoscopy. 1995; 27:171–7. doi: 10.1055/s-2007-1005657.

Natsugoe S, Yoshinaka H, Shimada M, et al. Number of lymph node metastases determined by presurgical ultrasound and endoscopic ultrasound is related to prognosis in patients with esophageal carcinoma. Ann Surg. 2001;234:613–18. doi: 10.1097/00000658-200111000-00005.

Chen J, Xu R, Hunt GC, et al. Influence of the number of malignant regional lymph nodes detected by endoscopic ultrasonography on survival stratification in esophageal adenocarcinoma. Clin Gastroenterol Hepatol. 2006;4:573–9. doi: 10.1016/j.cgh.2006.01.006.

Twine CP, Roberts SA, Rawlinson CE, et al. Prognostic significance of the endoscopic ultrasound defined lymph node metastasis count in esophageal cancer. Dis Esophagus. 2010;23:652–9. doi: 10.1111/j.1442-2050.2010.01072.x.

Li Z, Rice TW. Diagnosis and staging of cancer of the esophagus and esophagogastric junction. Surg Clin North Am. 2012;92:1105–26. doi: 10.1016/j.suc.2012.07.010.

Luketich JD, Friedman DM, Weigel TL, et al. Evaluation of distant metastases in esophageal cancer: 100 consecutive positron emission tomography scans. Ann Thorac Surg. 1999;68:1133–6; discussion 1136–7.

Brierley J, Gospodarowicz MK, Wittekind C, editors. TNM classification of malignant tumours. 8th ed. Chichester, West Sussex: John Wiley & Sons, Inc.; 2017.

The Royal College of Pathologists. Dataset for the histopathological reporting of oesophageal carcinoma. 2nd ed. London: The Royal College of Pathologists; 2007.

College of American Pathologists. Protocol for the examination of specimens from patients with carcinoma of the oesophagus. Northfield: College of American Pathologists; 2009.

Javidfar J, Speicher PJ, Hartwig MG, et al. Impact of positive margins on survival in patients undergoing esophagogastrectomy for esophageal cancer. Ann Thorac Surg. 2016;101:1060–7. doi: 10.1016/j.athoracsur.2015.09.005.

Liu X, Rice TW, Xiao SY, et al. Diagnostic problems during esophageal and gastric surgery. In: Marchevsky AM, Balzer BL, Abdul-Karim FW, editors. Intraoperative consultation. Philadelphia: Elsevier; 2015. p. 154–68.

Rizk NP, Ishwaran H, Rice TW, et al. Optimum lymphadenectomy for esophageal cancer. Ann Surg. 2010;251:46–50. doi: 10.1097/SLA.0b013e3181b2f6ee.

Shaheen NJ, Falk GW, Iyer PG, et al. ACG clinical guideline: Diagnosis and management of Barrett's esophagus. Am J Gastroenterol. 2016;111:30–50; quiz 51. doi: 10.1038/ajg.2015.322.

Lewis JT, Wang KK, Abraham SC. Muscularis mucosae duplication and the musculo-fibrous anomaly in endoscopic mucosal resections for Barrett esophagus: Implications for staging of adenocarcinoma. Am J Surg Pathol. 2008;32:566–71. doi: 10.1097/PAS.0b013e31815bf8c7.

Koen Talsma A, Shapiro J, Looman CW, et al. Lymph node retrieval during esophagectomy with and without neoadjuvant chemoradiotherapy: Prognostic and therapeutic impact on survival. Ann Surg. 2014;260:786–92; discussion 792–3. doi: 10.1097/SLA.0000000000000965.

Chang F, Deere H, Mahadeva U, et al. Histopathologic examination and reporting of esophageal carcinomas following preoperative neoadjuvant therapy: Practical guidelines and current issues. Am J Clin Pathol. 2008;129:252–62. doi: 10.1309/CCR3QN4874YJDJJ7.

Wu TT, Chirieac LR, Abraham SC, et al. Excellent interobserver agreement on grading the extent of residual carcinoma after preoperative chemoradiation in esophageal and esophagogastric junction carcinoma: A reliable predictor for patient outcome. Am J Surg Pathol. 2007;31:58–64. doi: 10.1097/01.pas.0000213312.36306.cc.

Hornick JL, Farraye FA, Odze RD. Prevalence and significance of prominent mucin pools in the esophagus post neoadjuvant chemoradiotherapy for Barrett's-associated adenocarcinoma. Am J Surg Pathol. 2006;30:28–35. doi: 10.1097/01.pas.0000174011.29816.fa.

Mandard AM, Dalibard F, Mandard JC, et al. Pathologic assessment of tumor regression after preoperative chemoradiotherapy of esophageal carcinoma: Clinicopathologic correlations. Cancer. 1994;73:2680–6. doi: 10.1002/1097-0142(19940601)73:11<2680::AID-CNCR2820731105>3.0.CO;2-C.

Ryan R, Gibbons D, Hyland JM, et al. Pathological response following long-course neoadjuvant chemoradiotherapy for locally advanced rectal cancer. Histopathology. 2005;47:141–6. doi: 10.1111/j.1365-2559.2005.02176.x.

Burt BM, Groth SS, Sada YH, et al. Utility of adjuvant chemotherapy after neoadjuvant chemoradiation and esophagectomy for esophageal cancer. Ann Surg. 2016. [Epub ahead of print]. doi: 10.1097/SLA.0000000000001954.

Chapter 5

Signs and Symptoms of Esophageal Cancer

5.1 GENERAL SIGNS AND SYMPTOMS OF ESOPHAGEAL PATHOLOGIES

A strictly taken anamnesis is very important in the correct diagnosis of esophageal diseases, including esophageal cancer. Among the most frequent signs we can mention:

5.1.1 Dysphagia

It can be functional and mechanical. A functional dysphagia is encountered when the disorder is of the central neuromuscular type, with swallowing problems from the level of the oral cavity, pharynx to the end of the esophagus. Mechanical dysphagia is caused by mechanical obstruction of transit both by a disease of the esophagus itself or by an external compressive mass. Functional neuromuscular dysphagia has a fundamental difference from organic dysphagia due to the fact that it has a slower progression and paradoxically begins with a difficulty of swallowing liquids and then solid foods. Mechanical dysphagia has a faster progression due to the difficulty in swallowing solid foods initially, to continue until the inability to pass even liquids.

5.1.2 Pyrosis

Otherwise, the retrosternal burning sensation is a typical sign caused by the regurgitation of acidic stomach contents into the esophagus.

5.1.3 Thoracic Pain

Progressive damage to the layers of the esophagus can be accompanied by chest pain, which requires differentiation with other diseases such as

DOI: 10.1201/9781003497547-5

acute coronary syndrome, aortic dissection, pulmonary thromboembolism, pneumothorax, etc.

5.1.4 Regurgitation

Return of gastric or esophageal contents. It can be accompanied by belching and heartburn. To judge the level of occlusion, the nature of the returned material, whether it is undigested or partially digested food and whether there is bile present, must be taken into consideration.

5.1.5 Emesis

Vomiting is the reflex emission of gastric contents from the activation of the stomach and abdomen muscles, often due to poisoning or indigestion. Voluminous or repeated vomiting can cause a rupture of the esophagus in the mediastinum (Boerhave syndrome) or a tear of the stomach at the level of the cardia, which is also accompanied by hematemesis (Mallory-Weiss syndrome).

5.2 SIGNS AND SYMPTOMS OF BENIGN TUMORS OF THE ESOPHAGUS

Benign tumors of the esophagus such as: leiomyomas, adenomatous polyps, cysts, neurofibromas, lymphangiomas, and hemangiomas have been mentioned in the previous chapters. Often these tumors are diagnosed incidentally during fibrogastro-duodenoscopy or CT scan and do not present clinical signs. An increase in the size of these tumors over 2 cm may present dysphagia.

5.3 SIGNS AND SYMPTOMS OF MALIGNANT TUMORS OF THE ESOPHAGUS

The two main types of esophageal cancer are adenocarcinoma and squamous cell carcinoma. According to the way of their macroscopic development, they can be of infiltrative, vegetative, and ulcerative forms.

The infiltrative form causes narrowing of the lumen of the esophagus and rigidity, and as a result organic type dysphagia and pain during swallowing, odynophagia.

Difficulty swallowing food causes weight loss and anorexia.

The progression of dysphagia with narrowing of the lumen continues with the inability to pass fluids up to complete and sialorrhea aphagia.

Rapid infiltration of the layers of the esophagus' surrounding structures can cause retrosternal and subscapular pain.

Involvement of the recurrent laryngeal nerve manifests with dysphonia, while involvement of the cervical ganglia may present Horner's syndrome (miosis, ptosis, enophthalmos, and anhidrosis). An affected phrenic nerve can be associated with hiccups.

Fistulization of the esophagus into the trachea or bronchi due to infiltration is associated with cough and pulmonary infections.

Infiltration of the aorta can be fatal with massive hemorrhage.

Rapid lymphnodal spread may make cervical adenopathy visible.

The vegetative form with endoluminal growth can ulcerate and show bleeding in the form of hematemesis, iron deficiency anemia, or melena.

BIBLIOGRAPHY

Cella DF, Tulsky DS, Gray G, et al. The functional assessment of cancer therapy scale: Development and validation of the general measure. J Clin Oncol. 1993;11(3):570–9. doi: 10.1200/JCO.1993.11.3.570.

Zeng H, Zheng R, Guo Y, et al. Cancer survival in China, 2003–2005: A population-based study. Int J Cancer. 2015;136(8):1921–30. doi: 10.1002/ijc.29227.

Zeng H, Zheng R, Guo Y. Analysis and prediction of esophageal cancer incidence trend in China. Chin J Prev Med. 2015;46(7):593–7.

Portenoy RK, Thaler HT, Kornblith AB, et al. Symptom prevalence, characteristics and distress in a cancer population. Qual Life Res. 1994;3(3):183–9. doi: 10.1007/BF00435383.

Chang VT, Hwang SS, Feuerman M, et al. Symptom and quality of life survey of medical oncology patients at a veterans affairs medical center: A role for symptom assessment. Cancer. 2000;88(5):1175–83. doi: 10.1002/(SICI)1097-0142(20000301)88:5<1175::AID-CNCR30>3.0.CO;2-N.

Darling GE. Quality of life in patients with esophageal cancer. Thorac Surg Clin. 2013;23(4):569–75. doi: 10.1016/j.thorsurg.2013.07.011.

Wang XS, Shi Q, Lu C, et al. Prognostic value of symptom burden for overall survival in patients receiving chemotherapy for advanced nonsmall cell lung cancer. Cancer. 2010;116(1):137–45.

Dodd MJ, Miaskowski C, Paul SM. Symptom clusters and their effect on the functional status of patients with cancer. Oncol Nurs Forum. 2001;28(3):465–70.

Kim HJ, McGuire DB, Tulman L, et al. Symptom clusters: Concept analysis and clinical implications for cancer nursing. Cancer Nurs. 2005;28(4):270–82. doi: 10.1097/00002820-200507000-00005.

Barsevick A. Defining the symptom cluster: How far have we come? Semin Oncol Nurs. 2016;32(4):334–50. doi: 10.1016/j.soncn.2016.08.001.

Miaskowski C, Barsevick A, Berger A, et al. Advancing symptom science through symptom cluster research: Expert panel proceedings and recommendations. J Natl Cancer Inst. 2017;109(4):djw253. doi: 10.1093/jnci/djw253.

Wikman A, Johar A, Lagergren P. Presence of symptom clusters in surgically treated patients with esophageal cancer: Implications for survival. Cancer. 2014;120(2):286–93. doi: 10.1002/cncr.28308.

Guo M, Wang C, Yin X, et al. Symptom clusters and related factors in oesophageal cancer patients 3 months after surgery. J Clin Nurs. 2019;28(19–20):3441–50. doi: 10.1111/jocn.14935.

Yu DS, Li PW, Chong SO. Symptom cluster among patients with advanced heart failure: A review of its manifestations and impacts on health outcomes. Curr Opin Support Palliat Care. 2018;12(1):16–24. doi: 10.1097/SPC.0000000000000316.

Gottlieb BH, Bergen AE. Social support concepts and measures. J Psychosom Res. 2010;69(5):511–20. doi: 10.1016/j.jpsychores.2009.10.001.

Cohen S, Wills TA. Stress, social support, and the buffering hypothesis. Psychol Bull. 1985;98(2):310–57. doi: 10.1037/0033-2909.98.2.310.

Wang Y, Zhu L, Yuan F, et al. The relationship between social support and quality of life: Evidence from a prospective study in Chinese patients with esophageal carcinoma. Iran J Public Health. 2015;44(12):1603–12.

Aydın Sayılan A, Demir Doğan M. Illness perception, perceived social support and quality of life in patients with diagnosis of cancer. Eur J Cancer Care (Engl). 2020;29(4):e13252. doi: 10.1111/ecc.13252.

Zhang Y, Cui C, Wang Y, et al. Effects of stigma, hope and social support on quality of life among Chinese patients diagnosed with oral cancer: A cross-sectional study. Health Qual Life Outcomes. 2020;18(1):112. doi: 10.1186/s12955-020-01353-9.

Chapter 6

Diagnosis of Esophageal Cancer

6.1 RADIOGRAPHY WITH ORAL CONTRAST

In order to get a better view of the esophagus and stomach, an oral contrast imaging examination is often performed, which the patient drinks and then undergoes evaluation. It should be noted that its sensitivity varies from the lowest to the highest, respectively, for non-invasive and invasive forms.

The limitations of this examination have been increasing over time and with the advancement of technologies in the field of medicine, losing to some extent the great importance it had, and being used mostly in establishing diagnoses of functional pathologies of the esophagus, achalasia, and esophageal diverticula.

Regardless of the above, the technique helps the operating surgeon to decide on the technique they will choose, the distance where they will perform the anastomosis, and also helps to establish the functionality of the anastomosis.

It remains an important technique in the detection of various fistulas, especially when combined with intravenous contrast.

6.2 ESOPHAGOGASTRO-DUODENOSCOPY AND BIOPSY

The so-called "gold standard", for the sole fact that the structural organization of this technique, with cameras and optical fibers, realizes a better visualization of the esophagus, stomach, or duodenum. The nature of the biopsy makes it a technique with almost 99% specificity and sensitivity for esophageal cancer.

In the field of Barrett's esophagitis, taking a biopsy throughout the mucosal extent enables endoscopic staging of adenocarcinoma, framing, and individualizing dysplastic and neoplastic areas.

DOI: 10.1201/9781003497547-6

Based on these biopsies, these lesions are divided into four classes:

1) Intestinal metaplasia without dysplasia.
2) Intestinal metaplasia with low-grade dysplasia.
3) Intestinal metaplasia with high-grade dysplasia.
4) Adenocarcinoma.

6.3   ECHOENDOSCOPY

The EUS technique enables the identification and study of the layers of the esophagus, making it possible to differentiate between lesions extending toward the muscular layer and confined lesions.

The technique, which is a bridge between endoscopic and ultrasound imaging, in addition to providing information on lymphnodal stations and their status, also provides information on resectability, helping the surgeon to make the right decision for the patient.

There are two types of endoscopic probes:

1) Those that allow the identification of the five layers of the esophagus and that use frequencies of 5–10 Hz.
2) And those that give a better wall resolution, highlighting nine layers, using 15–20 Hz frequencies.

In practice, the use of these probes has three advantages:

1) Differentiates lesions that are intramucosal from those that have affected the submucosa.
2) Mini probes, being mentioned as innovative techniques, perform mucosectomy with lower risks.
3) Verification of the depth in cases of mucosectomy.

6.4   MAGNIFYING CHROMOENDOSCOPY

It represents the technique which, by using a pigment, makes it possible to obtain information in cases where a biopsy has been taken in that area or when the area has been marked for resection. The use of colorants, in addition to the above benefits, also shows the affected lymph nodes, this is a consequence of the previous absorption of the stains by the tumor cells.

The dyes are different, starting with 1) vital dyes (Lugol, methylene blue), 2) contrast dyes, performing mucosal staining among which we mention acetic acid, 3) reactive dyes, which are characterized by their reaction to mucosal pH (phenol red), and 4) colorants such as tattoos that color the location of the injection, methylene blue is the main representative.

In achieving an accurate diagnosis, high-resolution endoscopes are also used which enlarge the image, often combined with acetic acid, achieving a precision in the diagnosis of esophageal cancer up to 92%.

It is precisely the development of these techniques that has made possible the morphological and vascular study, realizing the fine individualization of the mucosa and the precision of taking the biopsy.

Classification of the mucosal surface is a consequence of this technique to enlarge the mucosa. In this way we mention five classes: circular pattern, linear pattern, elongated ovular pattern, tubular pattern, and villous pattern.

The last three patterns are often associated with Barrett's intestinal metaplasia, while the tubular and villous patterns are associated with high-grade dysplasia.

6.5   CT SCANNER

Tomography is the other technique used in the detection and staging of esophageal cancer, in contrast to the PET scanner, it has a low sensitivity in detecting distant metastases. But the combination of both PET scanners on one hand, as well as thoraco-abdominal CT on the other hand, will give us a more detailed picture for the staging of esophageal cancer, distant metastases, as well as the description of the aorta, lymphadenopathy, or tracheobronchial infiltration.

6.6   MAGNETIC RESONANCE

Based on many resources, its difference with the technique mentioned previously is not very significant, even in some studies a low sensitivity is clearly shown, especially in pulmonary metastases. This is the reason that even in our practice at QSUT we use the scanner more, the use of which is limited only in cases of contraindication.

6.7   FIBRO-BRONCHOSCOPY

Since it is a technique that provides detailed information on the state of the respiratory tract, whether they have been infiltrated or not, whether their walls are rigid or not, it finds use and is one of the preferred techniques in cancer staging with position in the upper one-third of the esophagus to rule out tracheo-bronchial infiltration. Evidence of different vegetations indicates taking biopsies giving its own contribution to cancer staging.

6.8 PET AND PET SCANNER

It is described as a technique with a high reliability in the staging of advanced esophageal cancer, a high sensitivity in the staging of the tumor before the intervention, but no other element is evidenced that has advantages over standard techniques such as scanning or resonance.

It has an important role in evidencing the efficiency of chemotherapy, or tumor downstaging, in cases where we are before the intervention because it best studies bone metastases.

However, the role of the scanner in cancer staging is not diminished by the PET scanner, due to the fact that the latter gives us less information about the primary tumor, pulmonary, or hepatic metastases.

6.9 ENT EXAMINATION

The purpose of performing an ENT examination is to differentiate a primary tumor of the esophagus from that of the larynx or vocal cords, and to see infiltration of the vocal cords. Screening is preferred for squamous cell carcinoma.

6.10 NECK ULTRASOUND

For the study of metastatic supraclavicular and latero-cervical lymphadenopathy, it noted that the realization of ultrasound in these regions has resulted in an increase in sensitivity and specificity in conjunction with the scanner or PET scanner.

It is mostly used in lesions of the cervical and thoracic esophagus, making it possible to obtain a biopsy under the ultrasound regime.

BIBLIOGRAPHY

Sjoquist KM, Smithers BM, Burmeister BH, Survival after neoadjuvant chemotherapy or chemoradiotherapy for resectable oesophageal carcinoma: An updated meta-analysis. Lancet Oncol. 2011;11:671–91.

Pennathur A, Luketich JD, Ward J, et al. Long-term results of a phase II trial of neoadjuvant chemotherapy followed by esophagectomy for locally advanced esophageal neoplasm. Ann Thorac Surg. 2008 Jun;86(6):1930–5; discussion 1935–7. doi: 10.1016/j.athoracsur.2008.01.097. PMID: 18498697.

Clavien PA, de Oliveira ML, Barkun J, et al. The Clavien-Dindo classification of surgical complications: Five-year experience. Ann Surg. 2009;251:186–95.

Kumagai K, Rouvelas I, Tsai JA, et al. Meta-analysis of postoperative morbidity and perioperative mortality in patients receiving neoadjuvant chemotherapy or chemoradiotherapy for resectable oesophageal and gastro-oesophageal junctional cancers. Br J Surg. 2014;101:325–37.

Al-Sukhni E, Attwood K, Gabriel E, et al. No survival difference with neoadjuvant chemoradiotherapy compared with chemotherapy in resectable esophageal and gastroesophageal junction adenocarcinoma: Results from the national cancer data base. J Am Coll Surg. 2016;226:785–91.e1.

Luu TD, Force SD, Gaur P, et al. Neoadjuvant chemoradiation versus chemotherapy for patients undergoing esophagectomy for esophageal cancer. Ann Thorac Surg. 2008;85:1256–23; discussion 1225–4.

Wu AJ, Chang DT, Bosch WR, et al. Expert consensus contouring guidelines for IMRT in esophageal and gastroesophageal junction 13cancer. Int J Radiat Oncol Biol Phys. 2015 Jul 15;92(4):914–22. doi: 10.1026/.

Khan FM, Gerbi BJ. Treatment planning in radiation oncology. 3rd ed. Lippincott William & Wilkins/Wolters Kluwer; 2012.

Donington JS, Deschamps C, Nichols FC III, et al. Preoperative chemoradiation therapy does not improve early survival after esophagectomy for patients with clinical stage III adenocarcinoma the esophagus. Ann Thorac Surg. 2004;76:1196–9.

Chapter 7

Operative Techniques and Lymphatic Curage

In the last five years, I have had about 19 cases a year with carcinoma of the esophagus.

Of these, 94% resulted with squamous cell carcinoma and 6% with adenocarcinoma.

In 86% of cases, the patients started the treatment with the placement of a feeding jejunostomy and underwent the full cycle of radiotherapy accompanied by several chemotherapy sessions. Forty days after the end of chemotherapy, the patients underwent surgical resection.

In almost all cases I used the right thoracotomy, and only in four cases the left thoracotomy was used. As the most ideal approach to the thoracic esophagus I prefer the right thoracotomy, despite the best exposure of the lower esophagus is in the left thoracotomy.

In cases where the carcinoma is located in the lower one-third of the esophagus, I always start with the abdominal phase, and in cases where the carcinoma is located in the middle and upper part, I always start with a right thoracotomy. This is because we can accurately determine the operability of the patient.

In the management of esophageal carcinoma, two aspects are equally important, resection and reconstruction of the esophagus, so both moments deserve maximum attention. Inadequate resection would not achieve the goal of the operation, on the other hand, an unnecessary resection increases morbidity and mortality.

Another very important aspect in the management of esophageal carcinoma is lymphatic drainage. I am simplifying the lymphatic stations into seven regions:

- Neck region.
- Superior mediastinal region.
- Middle mediastinum region.
- Lower mediastinal region.

DOI: 10.1201/9781003497547-7

- Celiac trunk region.
- Curvatura major ventriculi region.
- Hepato-duodenal ligament region.

7.1 THORACIC PHASE

The patient is positioned laterally in the left lateral decubitus, the right arm is raised up and rests on the fixator, while the left arm is extended. Two sponge pads are placed under the chest to elevate it.

The incision begins in the fifth intercostal space from the border of the sternum to the lower corner of the shoulder. The fourth intercostal space can also be used depending on the location of the carcinoma. The incision continues with the electroscalpel. In the lower corner of the wound, the skin is separated and the latissimus dorsi muscle is exposed, which is carefully dissected and the serratus anterior muscle is exposed. The serratus anterior muscle is then cut with an electroscalpel and the intercostal muscles are reached.

The parasternal plexus containing the mammary artery and vein is cut and ligated. The intercostal muscles are cut with an electroscalpel along the superior costal margin.

After this action, the thorax is entered, the lungs are deflated with the help of the anesthesiologist after the intubation has been done selectively with the Carlens endotracheal tube. The automatic divaricator is placed between the ribs and the operative field is expanded by rotating the lever of the automatic divaricator (see Figure 7.1).

Adhesions of the pleura are carefully studied if there are any, but we must avoid unnecessary extrapleural dissection as they cause hemorrhage and complicate the situation. Pneumonia should be treated delicately, as we may have postoperative complications that endanger the patient's progress.

The next step is to assess the stage of the carcinoma, to decide whether it is operable or not, but it is difficult to determine from the beginning until the mediastinal dissection is performed, which gives us a more accurate picture of the patient's operability.

The mediastinal dissection is started from top to bottom. The right laryngeal nerve is identified and the lymphatic glands around it are carefully prepared as they pass close to the right subclavian artery. We must be very cautious even after identifying the laryngeal nerve around the subclavian artery in order not to damage this artery.

The pleura near the superior vena cava is incised and the right paratracheal lymph nodes between the trachea and the vein are resected. The upper limit of the gyration between the trachea and the superior vena cava

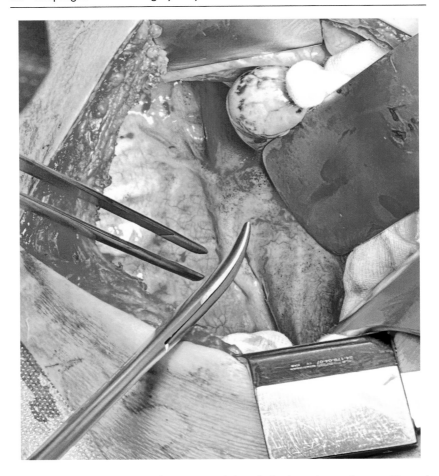

Figure 7.1 Lung retraction and exposure of the whole thoracic esophagus—General Surgery QSUT.

is achieved by visualizing the brachiocephalic artery, precisely the curage at this level is necessary since these glands often contain metastases.

Dissection continues along the vagus nerve and brachiocephalic artery. It continues with the preparation, cutting, and suturing of the two branches of the arch of the azygos vein (see Figure 7.2). Lymphatic dissection is performed at this level and dissection is continued in the region of the bifurcation of the trachea and the pulmonary hilus.

The pulmonary branches of the vagus and the bronchial artery are identified and preserved. Between the pericardium and the esophagus, exactly at the level of the lower pulmonary vein, we enter an avascular

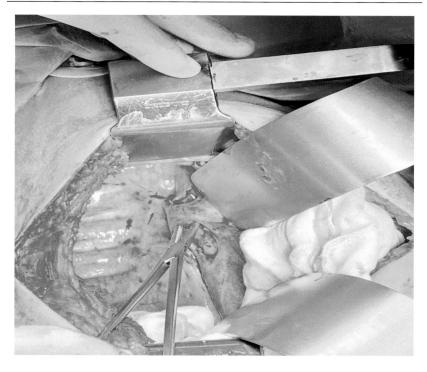

Figure 7.2 **Azygos vein dissection—General Surgery QSUT.**

plane and remove the lymph nodes of the bifurcation of the trachea and the lymph nodes of the carina.

The thoracic duct is easily identified, where many lymph glands are present, which are removed together with the duct. Care must be taken with the surrounding small ducts in order to ligate them as they can cause chylothorax.

It continues downward with the diaphragmatic glands and to the anterior part of the esophagus.

By keeping the esophagus in traction, its separation from the arch of the aorta, as well as an adequate control of hemostasis, is carried out carefully, then the descending aorta is prepared (as in Figure 7.3).

The next step is to cut the esophagus (see Figure 7.4). The upper limit of the tumor is determined and in the case of squamous carcinoma, the distance of the esophagus cut above the tumor is from 5–7 cm, and according to some authors up to 10 cm.

Whereas in adenocarcinomas, the upper limit is 3 cm. These resection limits are postulates that must always be respected.

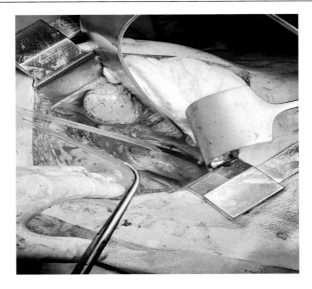

Figure 7.3 Passing a loop around the normal esophagus—General Surgery QSUT.

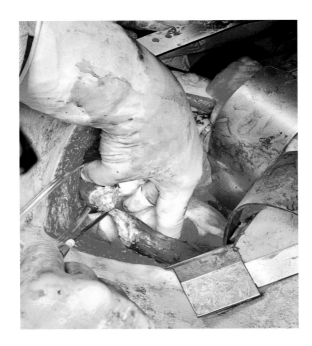

Figure 7.4 Esophageal resection—General Surgery QSUT.

7.2 ABDOMINAL PHASE

The patient turns decubitus dorsalis. A median incision is made from the xiphoid process to just below the umbilicus (see Figure 7.5). The peritoneal cavity is opened and a check is made of all the abdominal organs (see Figure 7.6).

It begins with the dissection of the greater omentum exactly along its insertion in the transverse colon, the omental bursa is entered, and the separation of the omentum from the lienal flexure of the colon continues.

The gastric vessels of the breves are carefully cut and ligated and the major curvature of the stomach is released from the spleen, also at the same time lymphatic drainage is done at the level of the lienal hilus.

It continues in the direction of the cardia of the stomach, releasing the phrenic-esophageal ligament, as a result, the stomach expands even more. The hepato-gastric ligament is cut and the lesser omental bursa is entered.

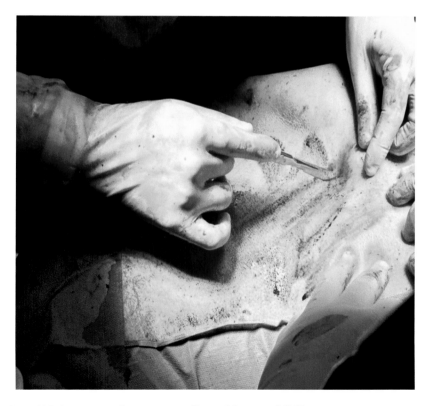

Figure 7.5 Superior midline incision—General Surgery QSUT.

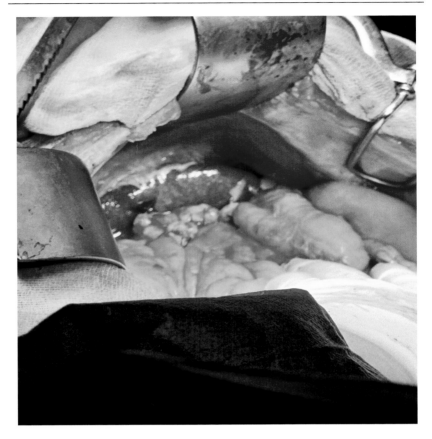

Figure 7.6 Exploring the abdominal cavity—General Surgery QSUT.

7.2.1   Abdominal Lymphatic Curage

The celiac trunk consisting of the hepatic artery, the left gastric artery, and the ileal artery is completely skeletonized by removing all surrounding lymph nodes.

It is continued with the curage at the level of the hepato-duodenal and retroduodenal ligament, after the Kocher maneuver is performed. Lymphatic curage is also done carefully along the right gastroepiploic artery, but without damaging it as it is the main source of blood supply for the gastric tube that will replace the esophagus.

After the celiac trunk is carefully prepared by performing lymphatic drainage, the left gastric artery is cut and ligated, the preparation is continued at the level of the esophageal hiatus, and the entire stomach is excised along with the cut esophagus (as in Figure 7.7).

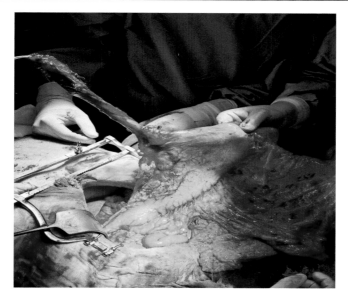

Figure 7.7 Stomach mobilization and thoracic esophagus extirpation—General Surgery QSUT.

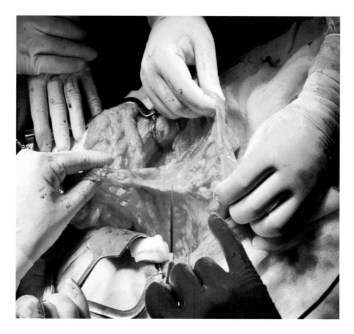

Figure 7.8 Division of omentum majus from the hepatic flexure of colon—General Surgery QSUT.

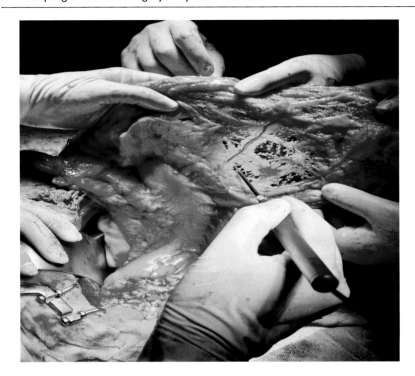

Figure 7.9 Resection of omentum majus, preserving the right gastroepiploic vessels—
General Surgery QSUT.

The operation continues with the separation of the omentum majus from the hepatic flexure of the colon (as in Figure 7.8), and throughout the preparation we will pay attention and be careful not to damage the right gastric artery.

Next, we continue with the Kochering of the duodenum, which starts from the pylorus to D3, also luxating D3. It is very important to luxate the duodenum as much as possible, as it facilitates the procedure for both intrathoracic and cervical anastomosis.

The omentum is carefully resected along the entire length of the major curvature while strictly maintaining the right gastric artery, damage to each would change the procedure of the intervention (see Figure 7.9).

After that comes the most important moment of the operation, the preparation of the stomach for anastomosis. Depending on the surgical procedure to be used, the stomach is cut creating the gastric tube that will be anastomosed with the esophagus. We use GIA to cut the stomach, but it can also be cut with a scalpel and sutured.

In the case of the Ivor-Lewis procedure, three or four GIAs may be used to create the gastric tube which is loosely anastomosed to the thorax without tension.

The problem lies in the preparation of the stomach for anastomosis in the neck, the Akiyama or McKeown procedure, that is, esogastro-cervical anastomosis. The incision with GIA starts from 3 cm above the pylorus and continues with small incision steps, because the smaller the incision steps are, the more stomach tissue we gain, making the stomach tube as long as possible and a tension-free cervical anastomosis (see Figures 7.10 and 7.11).

The gastric tube should have a width of about 3.5 cm, because the blood supply to the fundus of the stomach is more adequate than in a narrower gastric tube (see Figure 7.12). This is precisely where one of the secrets of the successful implementation of the Aiyama procedure lies. After gastrectomy

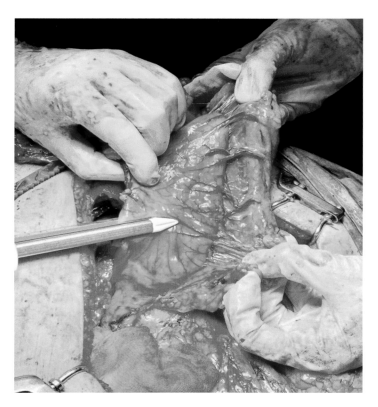

Figure 7.10 Starting to model the gastric tube—General Surgery QSUT.

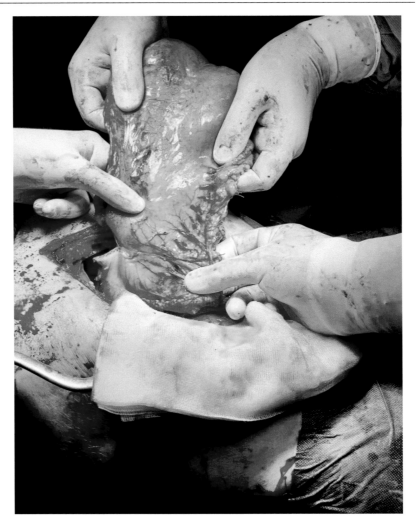

Figure 7.11 Starting the incision of the stomach 3 cm over the pylorus—General
Surgery QSUT.

with GIA, the margin of the gastric tube is sutured sero-serosally with vicryl
3.0 sutures.

The next step is the pyloroplasty, and in the case of the Ivor-Lewis
procedure, it continues with the execution of the intrathoracic eso-gastric
anastomosis. In cases of the Akiyama or McKeown procedure, the next
step is neck dissection (see Figure 7.13).

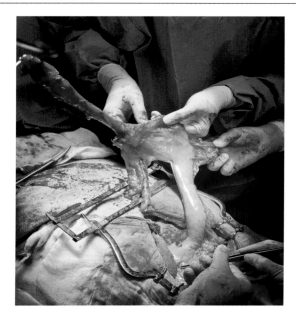

Figure 7.12 Preserving the width of the gastric tube, 3.5–4 cm—General Surgery QSUT.

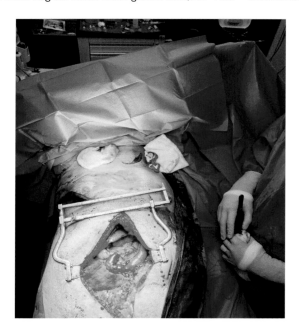

Figure 7.13 Three incisions: abdominal, thoracic, cervical—General Surgery QSUT.

7.3   CERVICAL PHASE

An incision is made parallel to the median margin of the left sternocleido-mastoid muscle in a length of about 7 cm, then it continues in the direction of the fossa jugularis (see Figure 7.14). Following the shape of a "V" the incision passes to the right. The anterior neck muscles are prepared, and the thyroid gland is entered. The middle thyroid vein and the inferior thyroid artery are cut and ligated, which makes it possible to luxate the thyroid, opening the operative field.

7.3.1   Cervical Lymphatic Curage

The cervical lymphatic gyrus is bounded medially by the esophagus, below the apical pleura, laterally by the laryngeal nerve, and above the medial thyroid vein. In the upper part of the clavicle, the areolar tissue of the omo-hyoid muscle is visible, containing lymph glands, which are removed (see Figure 7.15). Carefully visualize the thyrocervical trunk with its branches, the inferior thyroid artery, cervical artery, suprascapular artery together with the phrenic and vagus nerves. Lymphatic drainage is performed on

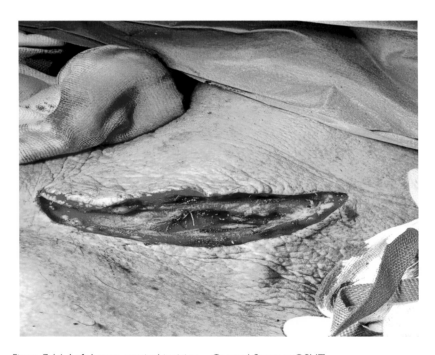

Figure 7.14 Left latero-cervical incision—General Surgery QSUT.

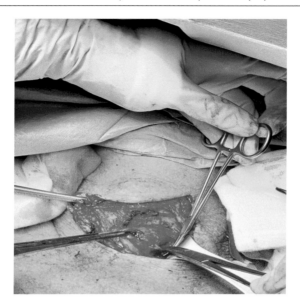

Figure 7.15 Preparing the omohyoid muscles, cervical lymphatic curage, luxation of the left thyroid lobe—General Surgery QSUT.

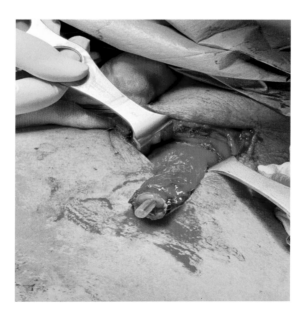

Figure 7.16 Luxation of esophageal stump—General Surgery QSUT.

the side of the internal jugular vein as well as the lymphatic chain of the laryngeal nerve.

After lymphatic curage is done at this level and the cervical esophagus is reached, which we begin to gently open so as not to damage the surrounding structures, and after we have checked the hemostasis, we take out the esophageal stump into the operative wound, which is ready for the reconstruction phase (see Figure 7.16).

7.3.1.1 The "Proper Margin" of the Proximal Esophageal Incision

Even today, the surgeon is often faced with the dilemma of how far the normal esophagus will be resected. The distance depends on the type and location of the carcinoma, therefore a careful and accurate intraoperative evaluation of the tumor is essential (see Figures 7.17 and 7.18). In cases where the location of the carcinoma is in the lower and middle one-third of the esophagus, the oncological cutting protocol must be respected, which indicates the resection of 5–7 cm of the normal esophagus. I am of the opinion that in cases of carcinomas located in the upper one-third, some compromises must be made, so we must not be too strict in respecting the distance according to the oncological protocol because a more mutilating operation will be needed, which also requires a laryngectomy, where primary importance in these the situation is to preserve the function of the larynx. However, this issue remains up for debate.

Despite the fact that at first glance the surgical margin appears free of tumor, there may be small intramural lesions covered with epithelium which are very difficult to diagnose with the naked eye. However, we are never sure that the remaining segment of the esophagus that will be anastomosed is healthy, although we respect the oncological protocol of the cutting margin of 5–7 cm.

Similarly, after preoperative esophageal resection, esophagitis with erosive changes appears. It is important to avoid anastomosis using damaged tissues, so that anastomotic stenoses do not occur. It is difficult to determine the diagnosis of esophagitis by looking at it from the outside, which makes cervical esophagotomy a necessity, in order to determine the exact limit of the esophageal resection.

It is precisely this boundary of the incision of the esophagus, that is, the remaining part of the proximal esophagus, that conditions the surgeon for the type of surgical procedure they will use, that is, they will perform the intrathoracic esophagogastric anastomosis, the Ivor-Lewis procedure or the cervical esophagogastric anastomosis, which includes the two procedures Akiyama and McKeown (see Figures 7.19 and 7.20). This procedure depends on the surgeon's preference. I personally prefer the Akiyama procedure, which I will explain in the following chapters.

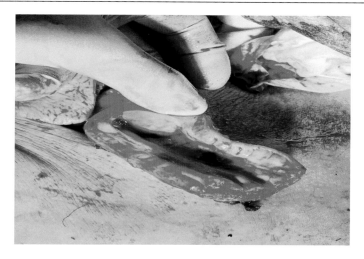

Figure 7.17 Internal inspection of esophageal stump—General Surgery QSUT.

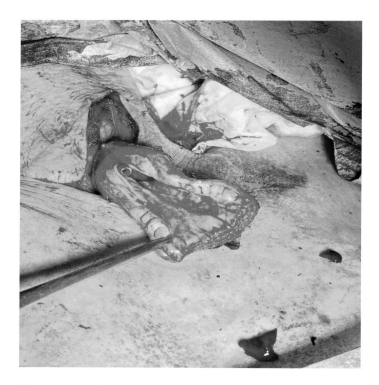

Figure 7.18 Longitudinal incision of the esophageal stump to clearly evidence healthy borders—General Surgery QSUT.

What I want to discuss now is my personal opinion about the division of the esophagus from the surgical point of view, I clarify with respect to the location of the carcinoma. In cases where the carcinoma is located in the lower one-third of the esophagus, the procedure to be used is Ivor-Lewis.

In cases where the carcinoma is located in the middle one-third, based on the oncological protocol of esophageal incision, the resection distance is 5–7 cm, or in some instances up to 10 cm, the remaining proximal part of the esophagus is short. The realization of an intrathoracic eso-gastric anastomosis is done under difficult technical conditions, which leads to an increased risk for the installation of anastomotic fistulas.

The opposite happens with cervical eso-gastric anastomosis where the surgeon feels more comfortable, and the management of anastomotic fistulas becomes easier and more adequate. Therefore, I am of the opinion that even in carcinomas located in the middle one-third of the esophagus, in order to avoid these technical difficulties and the increased occurrence of anastomotic fistulas, the chosen procedure should be Akiyama or McKeown, the surgeon chooses the procedure according to personal preference.

So anatomically the esophagus is divided into three upper, middle, and lower parts, while surgically it is divided into two parts, however this issue remains for discussion.

7.3.1.1.1   Intrathoracic Eso-Gastric Anastomosis

In the Ivor-Lewis procedure, the edges of the esophagus are processed, which are cut a little to see if their vascularization is good or not. If a poor vascularization of the edges of the esophagus that will be anastomosed is observed, then the incision of the esophagus is continued above until the vascularization is sufficient. The anastomosis can be performed manually or using a circular stapler with a diameter of 25 mm (see Figure 7.21).

7.3.1.1.2   Manual Anastomosis

We widen the esophageal hiatus by cutting the crus of the diaphragm and inserting the prepared stomach in the form of a tube along the posterior mediastinum. We verify that the stomach comes without tension and without torsion, which on the contrary will bring severe complications.

An incision is made in the anterior wall of the stomach and the eso-gastric anastomosis is performed with special 3/0 vicryl threads, suturing the posterior margin first and then the anterior margin. A nasogastric tube is passed and left approximately 4 cm above the pyloroplasty level.

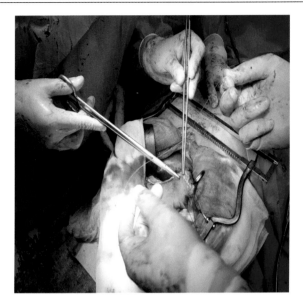

Figure 7.19 Preparing the stomach for intrathoracic anastomosis. Ivor-Lewis procedure—General Surgery QSUT.

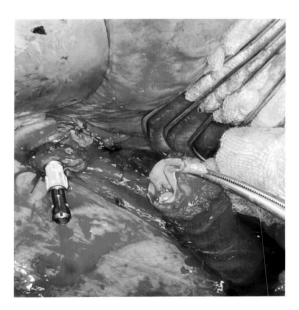

Figure 7.20 Mounting the stapler for an intrathoracic anastomosis—General Surgery QSUT.

The stomach is placed in the posterior mediastinum and fixed to the pleura with three to four sutures. The thoracic and abdominal cavity is lavaged and two drains are placed in each cavity. Both cavities are then closed.

7.3.1.1.3 Anastomosis with Stapler

A purse string suture with prolene is made around the esophagus, then the head of the stapler is placed inside the esophagus and the prolene is ligated. The rest of the stapler is inserted into the stomach and joined to the stapler head. After the stapler is fired, a "T" shaped GIA is used to close the stomach. The lips cut by the stapler are taken for biopsy.

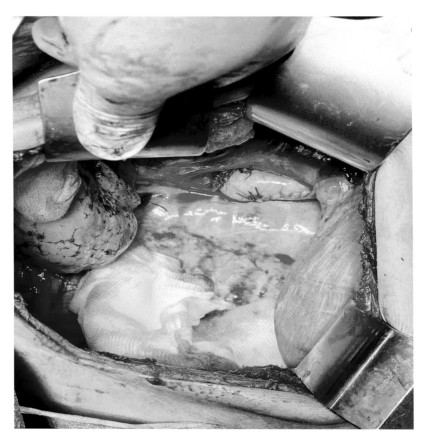

Figure 7.21 Eso-gastric intrathoracic anastomosis complete. Ivor-Lewis procedure—General Surgery QSUT.

7.3.1.1.4   Cervical Eso-Gastric Anastomosis

There are three ways to perform cervical anastomosis:

- Mediastinal presternal route.
- Anterior mediastinal tract.
- Posterior mediastinal tract.

In the early years of esophageal surgery, the presternal mediastinal route was preferred. Ignoring the unpleasant aesthetic aspect, this route had an important drawback—the distance from the abdomen to the neck compared to the other two mediastinal routes, being approximately 2 cm and 4 cm more distant than the retrosternal mediastinal and posterior mediastinal pathways, respectively.

So, we might have a lot of difficulties when positioning the stomach or colon in the cervical area. That is a reason why this path has been abandoned. I think nowadays this path is unsuitable.

The retrosternal pathway is easily created and starts from the xiphoid process (see Figure 7.22). At first, with two or three fingers it is prepared easily and carefully, pushed in the direction of the fossa jugularis. Then two

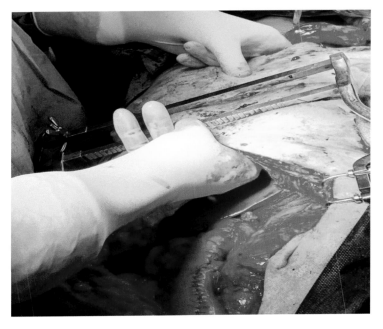

Figure 7.22 Digital retrosternal tunnelling—General Surgery QSUT.

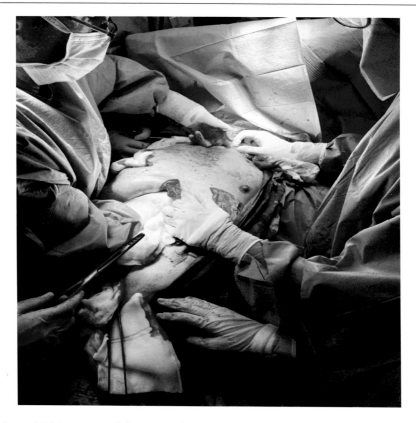

Figure 7.23 Insertion of the surgeon's forearm in the retrosternal region—General Surgery QSUT.

fingers are inserted in the same direction from the top downwards. This maneuver continues until both hands come together, creating a tunnel.

This tunnel should be widened until the surgeon's forearm is inserted (as in Figure 7.23).

Dilation of the tunnel is important as it reduces the bilateral pressure of the lungs on the gastric tube, which ensures better vascularization.

At the same time, the upper part of the retrosternal tunnel is expanded by partially cutting the sternothyroid muscle, which helps to reduce the pressure on the eso-gastric anastomosis. These constitute other secrets of this type of operation. In the anastomosis of this route, a transposition of the cervical esophagus occurs, deviating to the left from the natural position, which gives the patient a bad sensation during the passage of food, but it improves over time.

Above in the abdominal phase I described the preparation of the stomach for cervical anastomosis, since the stomach is more preferable to the colon, physiologically suitable, easier to prepare, and there is only one anastomosis. The use of the stomach as a substitute for the esophagus began with Gavriliu, Jianu, and their collaborators, and has been perfected year after year.

Even in my country in Albania, esophageal surgery has developed year after year with the passing of time, but we have not yet started to put laparoscopic procedures into use, while the ones that find use are classical surgery procedures.

Many esteemed professors have been and are dealing with this surgery, giving it a boost before esophageal surgery. From statistical data until 2019, the stomach as a substitute for the esophagus was used up to the thorax level, that is, intrathoracic eso-gastric anastomosis, the Ivor-Lewis procedure. In the cervical esophagus, in three cases, the anastomosis was performed using the colon as a substitute for the esophagus. This was the reason that gave me a big clue to study the use of the stomach to replace the resected esophagus, that is, to perform the Akiyama procedure for the first time in my country with interposition of the retrosternal stomach with cervical anastomosis. This became possible in March 2019, a case which I am presenting.

7.3.2 Presentation of Case I

The 62-year-old patient with the initials S.G. was known to the clinic two and a half months before. The patient undergoes a fibro-gastroscopy procedure, in which he is diagnosed with carcinoma of the esophagus between the upper and middle one-third of it. Through fibro-gastroscopy, a biopsy was taken, the result of which was squamous cell carcinoma.

In thoraco-abdominal CT with contrast, apart from the thickening of the esophagus in this region, no metastases in other organs or tumor infiltration in the surrounding regions around it was observed. The patient is taken into surgery and a feeding jejunostomy is performed.

The patient is further supplemented with radio-chemotherapy sessions, where respectively he undergoes 28 days of radiation and simultaneously three chemotherapy sessions. Thirty days after radio-chemotherapy the patient repeats a fibro-gastroscopy and a thoraco-abdominal CT. In fibro-gastroscopy, the tumor mass persisted, but reduced in size, while CT did not have data on metastases or surrounding infiltrations.

It is decided that the patient undergoes surgical intervention. Initially a right thoracotomy to assess its now objective operability. After careful preparation of the tumor from the surrounding structures, it was found to be resectable and the Akiyama procedure was performed, involving the placement of a gastric tube behind the sternum and the creation of an anastomosis between the cervical esophagus and the gastric tube.

On the third day following the surgery, the patient began receiving enteral nutrition through a jejunostomy.

On the seventh day after the surgery, an anastomosis check was conducted using gastrography.

Oral feeding was initiated on the eighth day post-surgery.

Finally, on the seventeenth day post-surgery, the patient was discharged from the hospital.

The next phase where care and attention should be paid is the positioning of the retrosternal stomach, already prepared in the form of a tube.

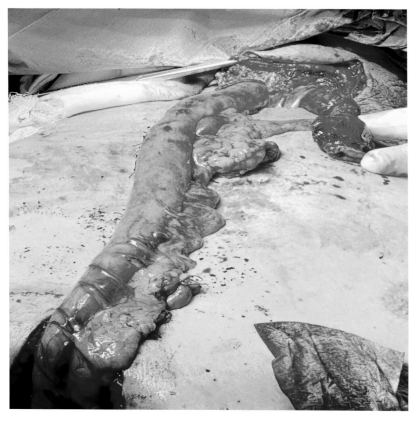

Figure 7.24 Measuring the gastric tube to avoid anastomotic tension—General Surgery QSUT.

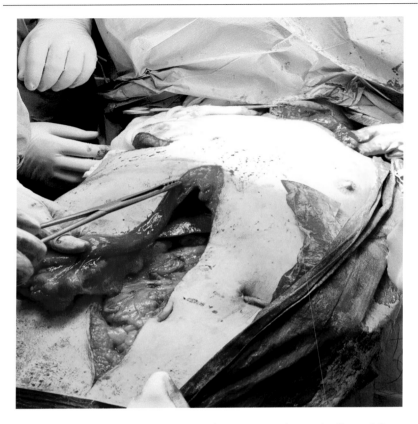

Figure 7.25 Passing of the gastric tube in the retrosternal tunnel—General Surgery QSUT.

The stomach should freely enter both the space at the level of the xiphoid process and at the level of the fossa jugularis, the latter being expanded by two fingers and cutting the sternothyroid muscle.

At the upper edge of the stomach, we sew a nasogastric tube (as in Figure 7.24). We insert the tube into the retrosternal tunnel from the xiphoid process and take it out into the jugular fossa, pull the already protruding tube into the cervical incision and fix the left hand at the level of the pylorus (see Figure 7.25).

We accompany the placement of the stomach in the retrosternal tunnel so that it does not twist, since its torsion is accompanied by torsion of the gastroepiploic vessels, which is fatal for the cervical eso-gastric anastomosis (as in Figure 7.26).

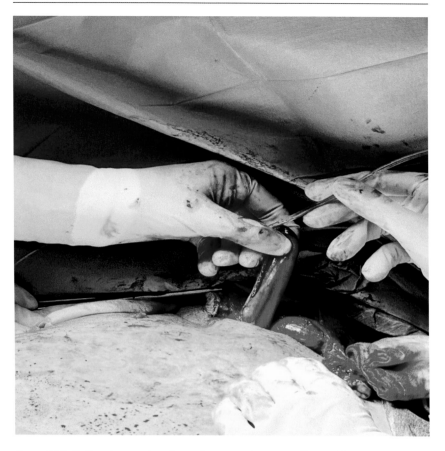

Figure 7.26 Pulling the gastric tube in the cervical region—General Surgery QSUT.

Cervical eso-gastric anastomosis can be performed with circular stapler, GIA 60 mm or manually using special sutures. Personally, in the nine cases of the Akiyama procedure that I performed, I used a circular stapler with a diameter of 25 mm to perform cervical eso-gastric anastomosis (see Figures 7.27, 7.28, 7.29, and 7.30). I fix the upper part of the gastric tube to the tissues around the neck, to reduce the tension at the level of the anastomosis and to prevent torsion of the gastric tube.

The cervical wound is closed, thoracic and abdominal drains are placed, and the respective wounds are closed. It should be noted that I have not placed a nasogastric tube.

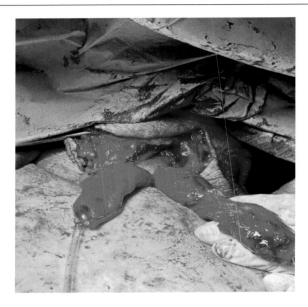

Figure 7.27 Exposing the gastric tube and esophageal stump ready for anastomosis—
General Surgery QSUT.

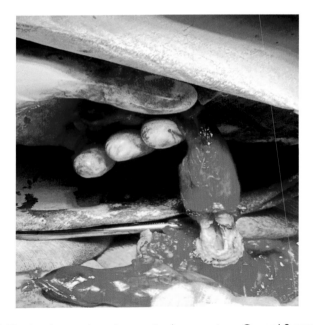

Figure 7.28 Cutting the esophageal stump in clear margins—General Surgery QSUT.

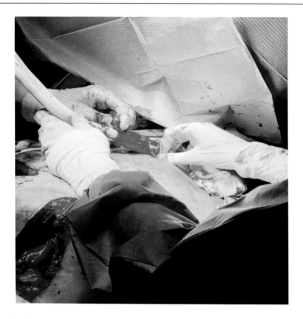

Figure 7.29 Circular stapler eso-gastric anastomosis—General Surgery QSUT.

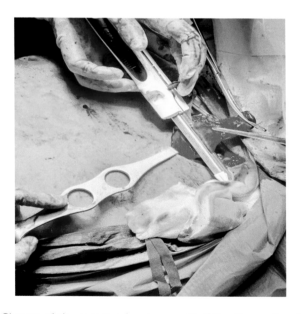

Figure 7.30 Closure of the gastric tube stump with GIA, after performing the eso-gastric anastomosis—General Surgery QSUT.

7.3.3 Overview of the Secrets of the Akiyama Procedure with Retrosternal Stomach Anastomosed to the Neck

- The cut starts 3 cm above the pylorus and continues with small steps, because this way we gain more length of the gastric tube (see Figures 7.31 and 7.32).
- The size of the gastric tube should be 3.5 cm (as in Figure 7.33) because the wider the tube, the better the vascularization of the upper part of the stomach is ensured, which is important for the anastomosis.
- Expansion of the retrosternal tunnel in the lower part until the surgeon's forearm is inserted (as in Figure 7.34), in order to reduce the pressure of the lungs on the stomach, while the expansion of the upper part of the tunnel is performed by cutting the sternothyroid muscle in order to reduce the pressure on the anastomosis.
- Fixation of the stomach with the surrounding cervical tissues reduces the tension on the anastomosis (see Figure 7.35).

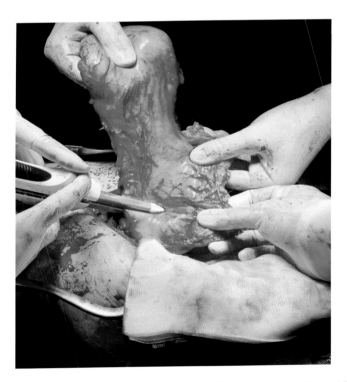

Figure 7.31 Starting of the stomach preparation for the gastric tube—General Surgery QSUT.

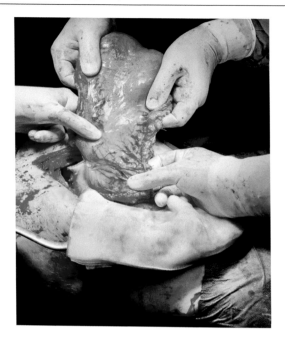

Figure 7.32 First cut with GIA, 3 cm over pylorus—General Surgery QSUT.

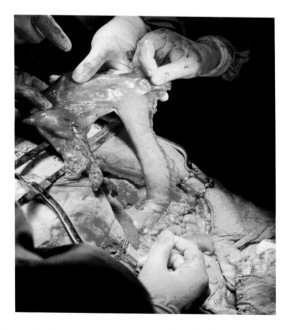

Figure 7.33 Preserving the width of the gastric tube 3.5–4 cm—General Surgery QSUT.

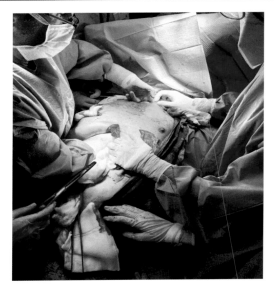

Figure 7.34 Retrosternal tunnel width measured with the surgeon's forearm—General Surgery QSUT.

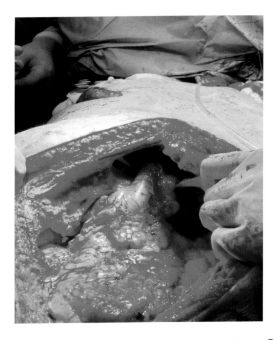

Figure 7.35 Lower fixation of the gastric tube to prevent torsion—General Surgery QSUT.

7.3.4   Cervical Eso-Colic Anastomosis

In eso-colic anastomosis, it is important to prepare the colon as best as possible preoperatively with a laxative substance.

The thoracic and cervical phase is the same as what we described above for esophagogastric anastomosis.

In the abdominal phase, it begins with the preparation of the transverse colon from the omentum majus and the stomach, and continues in the direction of the hepatic flexure, separating it from the duodenum.

In the next step, the lienal flexure of the colon is released and the vascular trunks are carefully inspected.

The colon is cut at the level of the lienal flexure, Riolan's arcade, and the middle of the transverse colon is also cut near the middle colic vessels, which is fanatically preserved as it will be the only vascular trunk that will supply this part of the digestive tract that will replace the esophagus.

The hepatic flexure of the colon is cut along with the vascular arcade. The side of the colon is closed at the level of the hepatic flexure and placed in a sterile bag which will accompany the colon in the retrosternal tunnel in order to avoid contamination of the mediastinum. Even at this stage, we will be careful and attentive to avoid torsion in order to maintain good vascularization.

The colon is placed in isoperistaltic position. After performing the eso-colic anastomosis, as in the eso-gastric anastomosis that we described above, two-layered colo-gastric and colo-colic anastomosis are performed.

* * *

After all this mental and physical fatigue of resection of the esophagus, the culminating moment is the anastomosis. It is precisely this that halves the life of the surgeon, whose mind rests on the anastomosis, whether they did it correctly or not, until the days pass and the patient does the test with oral contrast. Dehiscence of the anastomosis comes as a result of inaccuracy in its implementation by the surgeon, or an unnecessary negligence at the time of its implementation. There is no other justification, in my opinion.

The pride or pessimism of the surgeon, the life or death of the patient depends on the precise implementation of the anastomosis protocol.

In esophageal surgery, the essential principles of anastomosis are the same as those of the entire digestive tract:

- Sufficient blood supply.
- Free tension in the anastomosis.
- Meticulous approximation of the edges of the epithelium.
- Accurate layer-by-layer stitching.
- Non-irritating suture material.
- Meticulous mechanical stitching with stapler.

In both cases of stomach and colon replacement, pyloroplasty is performed at the end of the procedure (see Figure 7.36). In fact, I have
used it regularly in all esophageal resections, although there are surgeons
who are not so fanatical about pyloroplasty. But I start from the fact
that during the resection of the esophagus, the vagal trunk is cut, which
slows down the emptying of the stomach, as a result, the pressure in the
anastomosis increases.

That's why I recommend routine pyloroplasty.

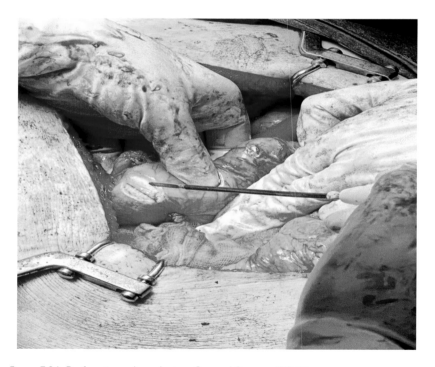

Figure 7.36 Performing pyloroplasty—General Surgery QSUT.

BIBLIOGRAPHY

Sjoquist KM, Smithers BM, Burmeister BH. Survival after neoadjuvant chemotherapy or chemoradiotherapy for resectable oesophageal carcinoma: An updated meta-analysis. Lancet Oncol. 2011;11:671–91.

Pennathur A, Luketich JD, Ward J, et al. Long-term results of a phase II trial of neoadjuvant chemotherapy followed by esophagectomy for locally advanced esophageal neoplasm. Ann Thorac Surg. 2008 Jun;86(6):1930–5; discussion 1935–7. doi: 10.1016/j. athoracsur.2008.01.097. PMID: 18498697.

Clavien PA, de Oliveira ML, Barkun J, et al. The Clavien-Dindo classification of surgical complications: Five-year experience. Ann Surg. 2009;251:186–95.

Kumagai K, Rouvelas I, Tsai JA, et al. Meta-analysis of postoperative morbidity and perioperative mortality in patients receiving neoadjuvant chemotherapy or chemoradiotherapy for resectable oesophageal and gastro-oesophageal junctional cancers. Br J Surg. 2014;101:325–37.

Al-Sukhni E, Attwood K, Gabriel E, et al. No survival difference with neoadjuvant chemoradiotherapy compared with chemotherapy in resectable esophageal and gastroesophageal junction adenocarcinoma: Results from the national cancer data base. J Am Coll Surg. 2016;226:785–91.e1.

Luu TD, Force SD, Gaur P, et al. Neoadjuvant chemoradiation versus chemotherapy for patients undergoing esophagectomy for esophageal cancer. Ann Thorac Surg. 2008;85:1256–23; discussion 1225–4.

Wu AJ, Chang DT, Bosch WR, et al. Expert consensus contouring guidelines for IMRT in esophageal and gastroesophageal junction 13cancer. Int J Radiat Oncol Biol Phys. 2015 Jul 15;92(4):914–22. doi: 10.1026/.

Khan FM, Gerbi BJ. Treatment planning in radiation oncology. 3rd ed. Lippincott William & Wilkins/Wolters Kluwer; 2012.

Donington JS, Deschamps C, Nichols FC III, et al. Preoperative chemoradiation therapy does not improve early survival after esophagectomy for patients with clinical stage III adenocarcinoma the esophagus. Ann Thorac Surg. 2004;76:1196–9.

Lin FC, Ferguson MK, Durkin AE. Induction therapy does not increase surgical morbidity after esophagectomy for cancer. Ann Thorac Surg. 2004; 77:1793–8.

Lee CH, Lee JM, Wu DC, et al. Carcinogenetic impact of alcohol intake on squamous cell carcinoma risk of the oesophagus in relation to tobacco smoking. Eur J Cancer 2007;44:1288–99.

Umar SB, Fleischer DE, Lee JM. Esophageal cancer: Epidemiology, pathogenesis and prevention. Nat Clin Pract Gastroenterol Hepatol. 2008;5:537–42.

Barrios E, De Stefani E, Fierro L. Black (air-cured) and blond (flue-cured) tobacco and cancer risk. III: Oesophageal cancer. Eur J Cancer. 1993; 29A:764–8.

Kristal A, Vaughan TL, Davis S, et al. Obesity, alcohol, and tobacco as risk factors for cancers of the esophagus and gastric cardia: Adenocarcinoma versus squamous cell carcinoma. Cancer Epidemiol Biomarkers Prev. 1995;4:86–93.

Silverman D, Brown LM, Hoover R, et al. Excess incidence of squamous cell esophageal cancer among US Black men: Role of social class and other risk factors. Am J Epidemiol. 2001;153:115–23.

Abnet CC, Mark SD. Prospective study of tooth loss and incident esophageal and gastric cancers in China. Cancer Causes Control. 2001;12:848–57.

Yang SJ, Wang HY, et al. Genetic polymorphisms of ADH2 and ALDH2 association with esophageal cancer risk in southwest China. World J Gastroenterol. 2007;13:576–76.

Risk JM, Garde J, et al. The tylosis esophageal cancer (TOC) locus: More than just a familial cancer gene. Dis Esophagus. 1999;12:178–9.

Poynton AR, O'Sullivan G. Carcinoma arising in familial Barrett's esophagus. Am J Gastroenterol. 1996;91:185.

Bollschweller E, Holscher AH, et al. Prognostic differences between early squamous cell and adenocarcinoma of the esophagus. Dis esophagus. 1997;10:178–83.

Edge SB, Compton CC. The American Joint Committee on Cancer: The 7th edition of the AJCC cancer staging manual and the future of TNM. Surg Oncol. 2010 Jun;17(6):1481–4.

Cameron AJ, Conio M, et al. Endoscopic treatment of high-grade dysplasia and early cancer in Barrett's esophagus: Review. Lancet Oncology. 2005:1–2.

Gossner L, Ell C, Mat A, et al. Endoscopic mucosal resection of early cancer high-grade dysplasia in Barrett's esophagus. Gastroenterol. 2000:670–9.

Kanao H, Tanaka S. Clinical significance of type V pit pattern subclassification in determining the depth of invasion of colorectal neoplasms. World J Gastroenterol. 2008 Jan;14:211–17.

Bonavina L, Incarbone R, Bona D, Peracchia A. Esophagectomy via laparoscopy and transmediastinal endodissection. J Laparoendosc Adv Surg Tech A. 2004;14:13–16.

Kunz S, Low DE, Schembre D, et al. Esofagectomy—it is not just mortality anymore: Standardized perioperative clinical pathways improve outcomes in patients with esophageal cancer. J Gastrointest Surg. 2007;11:1395–1402.

Orringer MB, Marshall B, Chang AC, et al. Two thousand transhiatal esophagectomies: Charging trends, lessons learned. Ann Surg. 2007 Sep;246(3):363–72; discussion 372–4. doi: 10.1097/SLA.0b013e31814697f2. PMID: 17717440; PMCID: PMC1959358.

Greenstein AJ, Little VR, Swanson SJ, et al. Effect of the number of lymphnodes sampled on prospective survival of lymph node negative esophageal cancer. Cancer. 2008 Mar 15;112(6):1239–46. doi: 10.1002/cncr.23309. PMID: 18224663.

Coda S, Oda I, Saito Y. EMR and ESD for early gastrointestinal cancers. In: Conio M, Siersema PD, Repici A, Ponchon T, editors. Endoscopic mucosal resection. Oxford: Blackwell Publishing; 2008. p. 185–98.

Ronellenfitsch U, Schwarzbach M, Hofheitz R, et al. Preoperative Cheo(radio) therapy versus primary surgery for gastroesophageal adenocarcinoma: Systematic review with meta-analysis combining individual patient and aggregate data. Eur J Cancer. 2013 Oct;49(15):3149–58. doi: 10.1016/j.ejca.2013.05.029. Epub 2013 Jun 22. PMID: 23800671.

Li X, Zhao LJ, Liu NB, et al. Feasibility and efficacy of concurrent chemo-radiotherapy in elderly patients with esophageal squamous carcinoma: A retrospective study of 116 cases from a single institution. Asian Pac J Cancer Prev. 2015;16(4):1463–9. doi: 10.7314/apjcp.2015.16.4.1463. PMID: 25743816.

Jenkinson AD, Lim J, Agrawl N, et al. Laparoscopic feeding jejunostomy in esophagogastric cancer. Surg Endosc. 2007. Evolué de l'oesophage thoraci-que: Anastomose oesogastrique au cou ou dans le thorax? Résultats tardifs d'une étude prospective "randomisée". Ann Chir. 1992;46:905–11.

Lam TCF, Fok M, Cheng SW, et al. Anastomotic complications after esopha-gectomy for cancer: A comparison of neck and chest anastomoses. J Thor Cardiovasc Surg. 1992;104:395–400.

Akiyama H, Tsurumaru M, Udagawa H, et al. Radical lymph node dissection for cancer of the thoracic oesophagus. Ann Surg. 1994;220:364–73.

Baba M, Aikou T, Yoshinaka H, et al. Long-term results of subtotal esophagec-tomy with three-field lymphadenectomy for carcinoma of the thoracic esophagus. Ann Surg. 1994;219:310–16.

Nishihira T, Hirayama K, Mori S. A prospective randomized trial of extended cervical and superior mediastinal lymphadenectomy for carcinoma of the thoracic esophagus. Am J Surg. 1998;175:47–51.

Hayes N, Shaw IH, Raimes SA, et al. Comparison of conventional Lewis-Tanner two-stage oesophagectomy with the synchronous two-team approach. Br J Surg. 1995;82:95–7.

Triboulet JP, Mariette C, Chevalier D, et al. Surgical management of carcinoma of the hypopharynx and cervical esophagus: Analysis of 209 cases. Arch Surg. 2001;136:1164–70.

Couraud L, Velly JF, Clerc P, et al. Experience of partial oesophagectomy in sur-gical treatment of lower and middle thoracic oesophageal cancer: From a follow-up of 366 cases. Eur J Cardiothorac Surg. 1989;3(2):99–103; discus-sion 104. doi: 10.1016/1010-7940(89)90085-7. PMID: 248334.

Cense HA, van Eijck CH, Tilanus HW. New insights in the lymphatic spread of oesophageal cancer and its implications for the extent of surgical resection. Best Pract Res Clin Gastroenterol. 2006;20(5):893–906. doi: 10.1016/j.bpg.2006.03.010. PMID: 16997168.

Bîrlă R, Iosif C, Mocanu A, et al. Long-term survival after eso-gastrectomy for esophagogastric junction adenocarcinoma–prospective study. Chirurgia (Bucur). 2008 Nov–Dec;103(6):635–42. PMID: 19274907 Romanian.

Pedrazzani C, Pasini F, Giacopuzzi S, et al. Surgical treatment of gasto-esophageal junction adenocarcinoma: Long-term results of a single Italian centre. G Chir. 2004 Oct;25(10):325–33. PMID: 15756954.

Stein HJ, Feith M, Siewert JR. Individualized surgical strategies for cancer of the esophagogastric junction. Ann Chir Gynaecol. 2000;89(3):191–8. PMID: 11079787.

Feith M, Stein HJ, Siewert JR. Adenocarcinoma of the esophagogastric junction: Surgical therapy based on 1602 consecutive resected patients. Surg Oncol Clin N Am. 2006 Oct;15(4):751–64. doi: 10.1016/j.soc.2006.07.015. PMID: 17030271.

Rüdiger Siewert J, Feith M, Werner M, et al. Adenocarcinoma of the esophagogastric junction: Results of surgical therapy based on anatomical/topographic classification in 1,002 consecutive patients. Ann Surg. 2000 Sep;232(3):353–61. doi: 10.1097/00000658-200009000-00007. PMID: 10973385.

Mönig SP, Schröder W, Beckurts KT, et al. Classification, diagnosis and surgical treatment of carcinomas of the gastroesophageal junction. Hepatogastroenterology. 2001 Sep–Oct;48(41):1231–7. PMID: 11677937.

Bai JG, Lv Y, Dang CX. Adenocarcinoma of the esophagogastric junction in China according to Siewert's classification. Jpn J Clin Oncol. 2006 Jun; 36(6):364–7. doi: 10.1093/jjco/hyl042. Epub 2006 Jun 9. PMID: 16766566.

McManus K, Anikin V, McGuigan J. Total thoracic oesophagectomy for oesophageal carcinoma: Has it been worth it? Eur J Cardiothorac Surg. 1999 Sep;16(3):261–5. doi: 10.1016/s1010-7940(99)00223-7. PMID: 10554840.

Maher M, Ali A, Qureshi H, et al. Transhiatal oesophagectomy for carcinoma oesophagus: Early experience. J Pak Med Assoc. 1991 Jun;41(6):129–31. PMID: 1895496.

Rindani R, Martin CJ, Cox MR. Transhiatal versus Ivor-Lewis oesophagectomy: Is there a difference? Aust N Z J Surg. 1999 Mar;69(3):187–94. doi: 10.1046/j.1440-1622.1999.01520.x. PMID: 10075357.

Omloo JM, Lagarde SM, Hulscher JB, et al. Extended transthoracic resection compared with limited transhiatal resection for adenocarcinoma of the mid/distal esophagus: Five-year survival of a randomized clinical trial. Ann Surg. 2007 Dec;246(6):992–1000; discussion 1000–1. doi: 10.1097/SLA.0b013e31815c4037. PMID: 18043101.

Peracchia A, Bonavina L, Via A, et al. Current trends in the surgical treatment of esophageal and cardia adenocarcinoma. J Exp Clin Cancer Res. 1999 Sep;18(3):289–94. PMID: 10606171.

Walther B, Johansson J, Johnsson F, et al. Cervical or thoracic anastomosis after esophageal resection and gastric tube reconstruction: A prospective randomized trial comparing sutured neck anastomosis with stapled intrathoracic anastomosis. Ann Surg. 2003 Dec;238(6):803–12; discussion 812–4. doi: 10.1097/01.sla.0000098624.04100.b1. PMID: 14631217.

Fok M, Wong J. Cancer of the oesophagus and gastric cardia: Standard oesophagectomy and anastomotic technique. Ann Chir Gynaecol. 1995; 84(2):179–83. PMID: 7574378.

Kimose HH, Lund O, Hasenkam JM, et al. Independent predictors of operative mortality and postoperative complications in surgically treated carcinomas of the oesophagus and cardia–is the aggressive surgical approach worthwhile? Acta Chir Scand. 1990 May;156(5):373–82. PMID: 1693462.

Svanes K, Stangeland L, Viste A, et al. Morbidity, ability to swallow, and survival, after oesophagectomy for cancer of the oesophagus and cardia. Eur J Surg. 1995 Sep;161(9):669–75. PMID: 8541426.

Jensen BM, Andersen KB. Surgical treatment of cancer of the esophagus and cardia. Ugeskr Laeger. 1998 Jul 27;160(31):4531–3. PMID: 9700310.

Sabanathan S, Eng J. Left thoracotomy approach for resection of carcinoma of the oesophagus and cardia. Ann Ital Chir. 1992 Jan–Feb;63(1):25–31. PMID: 1605442.

Kakeji Y, Takahashi A, Hasegawa H, et al. Surgical outcomes in gastroenterological surgery in Japan: Report of the National Clinical Database 2011–2018. Ann Gastroenterol Surg. 2020;4:250–74.

Takeuchi H, Miyata H, Gotoh M, et al. A risk model for esophagectomy using data of 5354 patients included in a Japanese nationwide web-based database. Ann Surg. 2014;260:259–66.

Chevallay M, Jung M, Chon SH, et al. Esophageal cancer surgery: Review of complications and their management. Ann N Y Acad Sci. 2020;1482:146–62.

Markar S, Gronnier C, Duhamel A, et al. The impact of severe anastomotic leak on long-term survival and cancer recurrence after surgical resection for esophageal malignancy. Ann Surg. 2015;262:972–80.

Jansen SM, de Bruin DM, van Berge Henegouwen MI, et al. Optical techniques for perfusion monitoring of the gastric tube after esophagectomy: A review of technologies and thresholds. Dis Esophagus. 2018;1:31.

Brinkmann S, Chang DH, Kuhr K, et al. Stenosis of the celiac trunk is associated with anastomotic leak after Ivor-Lewis esophagectomy. Dis Esophagus. 2019;1:32.

Tsunoda S, Obama K, Hisamori S, et al. Lower incidence of postoperative pulmonary complications following robot-assisted minimally invasive esophagectomy for esophageal cancer: Propensity score-matched comparison to conventional minimally invasive esophagectomy. Ann Surg Oncol. 2021;28:639–47.

Lainas P, Fuks D, Gaujoux S, et al. Preoperative imaging and prediction of oesophageal conduit necrosis after oesophagectomy for cancer. Br J Surg. 2017;104:1346–54.

Robba C, Cardim D, Sekhon M, et al. Transcranial doppler: A stethoscope for the brain-neurocritical care use. J Neurosci Res. 2018;96:720–30.

Noshiro H, Urata M, Ikeda O, et al. Invasive esophagectomy. Surgery. 2013;154:604–10.

Kim EN, Lamb K, Relles D, et al. Median arcuate ligament syndrome-review of this rare disease. JAMA Surg. 2016;151:471–7.

Horton KM, Talamini MA, Fishman EK. Median arcuate ligament syndrome: Evaluation with CT angiography. Radiographics. 2005;25:1177–82.

Liebermann-Meffert DM, Meier R, Siewert JR. Vascular anatomy of the gastric tube used for esophageal reconstruction. Ann Thorac Surg. 1992; 54:1110–5.

Lammerts RGM, van Det MJ, Geelkerken RH, et al. Risk-assessment of esophageal surgery: Diagnosis and treatment of celiac trunk stenosis. Thorac Cardiovasc Surg Rep. 2018;7:e21–3.

Kassis ES, Kosinski AS, Ross P Jr, et al. Predictors of anastomotic leak after esophagectomy: An analysis of the society of thoracic surgeons general thoracic database. Ann Thorac Surg 2013;96:1919–26.

Markar SR, Arya S, Karthikesalingam A, et al. Technical factors that affect anastomotic integrity following esophagectomy: Systematic review and meta-analysis. Ann Surg Oncol 2013;20:4274–81.

Schmidt HM, Gisbertz SS, Moons J, et al. Denning benchmarks for transthoracic esophagectomy: A multicenter analysis of total minimally invasive esophagectomy in low risk patients. Ann Surg. 2017;266:814–21.

Huang HT, Wang F, Shen L, et al. Clinical outcome of middle thoracic esophageal cancer with intrathoracic or cervical anastomosis. Thorac Cardiovasc Surg. 2015 Jun;63(4):328–34. doi: 10.1055/s-0034-1371509. Epub 2014 Apr 8. PMID: 24715527.

Wormald JC, Bennett J, van Leuven M, et al. Does the site of anastomosis for esophagectomy affect long-term quality of life? Dis Esophagus. 2016;29:93–8.

Akiyama S, Ito S, Sekiguchi H, et al. Preoperative embolization of gastric arteries for esophageal cancer. Surgery 1996;120:542–6.

Chapter 8

Results of Esophageal Surgery

Mortality	Number of patients/percentage
Intraoperative	0 deaths or 0%
Postoperative	6 cases of death or 6.1%

Complication	Number of patients/percentage
Eso-Gastric intrathoracic fistula	4 cases or 4%
Atelectasis and pulmonary thrombo-embolism	1 case or 1%
Chylothorax	1 case or 1%
Hemoperitoneum	1 case or 1%
Moderate hemothorax	1 case or 1%
Re-Interventions	3 cases or 3%

Chosen procedure	Number of patients/percentage
Ivor-Lewis procedure	90 cases or 90.9%
Akiyama procedure	9 cases or 9.1%. (no deaths or complications in all 9 cases)
Preoperative radio-chemotherapy	85 cases or 85.9%

Thoracic approach	Number of patients/percentage
Right thoracotomy	95 cases or 96%
Left thoracotomy	4 cases or 4%

Lymphatic curage performed and lymph nodes affected by malignance	Patients/percentage
Lymphatic curage	99 cases or 100%
Lymph nodes affected by malignance	42 cases or 42.4%

DOI: 10.1201/9781003497547-8

Chosen jejunostomy	Number of patients/percentage
Preoperative jejunostomy	81 cases or 81.8%
Intraoperative jejunostomy	18 cases or 18.2%

Hospital stay	16–18 days

8.1   WHY DID I USE THE CLASSIC SURGICAL APPROACH FOR THE IVOR-LEWIS PROCEDURE AND AKIYAMA PROCEDURE?

In my country, Albania, laparoscopy has entered en-masse in many types of operations of the digestive tract and has made great progress, but in esophageal surgery it is limited to achalasia or reflux procedures.

We have not yet reached esophagectomy with thoracoscopy, laparoscopy, or robotics as used in developed countries where esophageal surgery has reached its peak.

However, even today in the world there are many controversies in the management of esophageal cancer despite many clinical trials being conducted on a great difference in epidemiology and histology. There are many different options in the treatment of esophageal carcinoma and the best surgical access or extent of lymphatic drainage has not yet been determined.

Personally, I have rarely used the transhiatal route, especially in cases of carcinomas located in the lower one-third where I performed a superior polar resection, but in the case of tumor localization above, I think that we cannot visualize well the esophagus carcinoma, its extension, the regional infiltration.

Using classic thoracotomy surgery:

- A much clearer visualization of the tumor is obtained.
- An adequate lymphatic curage is performed, so important from an oncological point of view for a neoplasm.
- The of risk for anastomotic leaks decreases, the consequence of which is stenosis at this level.
- The risk of recurrence nerve damage decreases, this in cases of cervical anastomosis.

Of the advantages of the transhiatal route we mention:

- Reduction of pulmonary complications.
- Reduction of mortality since the operation takes a short time.

However, I am of the opinion that the surgeon chooses the path they know how to do best, no matter how long and difficult it may be, it is enough to strictly apply the oncological principles and most importantly to improve the patient's life.

8.2   THE ROLE OF JEJUNOSTOMY IN PATIENTS OPERATED ON WITH CARCINOMA OF THE ESOPHAGUS

I placed a jejunostomy in almost all patients.

Before performing the resection of the esophagus, in 81 cases, that is, in 81.8% of the patients, I placed a jejunostomy before these patients underwent the full cycle of radiotherapy and partial chemotherapy, three or four cycles. So, I was forced to have this procedure because during radiotherapy an edema of the part of the esophagus that is irradiated occurs and the patient cannot eat. Through the jejunostomy, we kept the patient's daily caloric intake at satisfactory levels.

In 18 cases, that is, in 18.2% of patients, I placed a jejunostomy during esophageal resection.

In 82% of the patients, on the third day after resection of the esophagus, I started enteral feeding, increasing the daily caloric intake, so necessary for these types of interventions and significantly improving their general condition.

I think that placing the jejunostomy and putting it into operation as early as possible has influenced the rehabilitation of postoperative patients until the patient starts to be fed regularly through the oral route.

I have read in the literature that some surgeons do not agree on the routine placement of a jejunostomy, as it carries many risk factors during its placement and use. I respect these opinions, but it has helped me a lot and I will continue to apply it.

8.2.1   Case Presentation

I am presenting the most difficult case that I have encountered in esophageal surgery, the technical and morbid difficulties it presented.

Patient in his 60s, male, with a deformity of the mandible and neck as a result of an intervention and radio-chemotherapy performed five years ago in the context of a tumor of the floor of the mouth.

The patient presents with high-grade dysphagia, significant weight loss. Fibro-gastroscopy results in a tumoral neoformation in the esophagus located 25 cm from the dental arcade, the biopsy of which shows squamous cell carcinoma. Contrast-enhanced thoraco-abdominal CT shows thickening of the esophagus between its middle and upper one-third, no surrounding infiltrations, no remote metastases.

I consulted the case with the radiotherapists and together we decided the standard procedure of jejunostomy, radio-chemotherapy, and finally the resection, whether it would be possible or not. The patient has a jejunostomy, completes the full cycle of radiotherapy and three cycles of chemotherapy.

On the 40th day after radio-chemotherapy, he was hospitalized and repeated fibro-gastroscopy and thoraco-abdominal CT control with IV contrast.

Despite the fact that after radiotherapy the patient started to eat, the tumor persisted in the fibroscope, the tomographic aspect remained the same, without regional infiltrations, no distant metastases. After the consultation, the decision for surgical intervention is made.

In the thoracic and abdominal phase there were no problems. In the cervical phase I encountered difficulties in its dissection as it had formed fibrosis from the radiation for the cancer of the floor of the mouth. Slowly and carefully, I was able to prepare and resect the esophagus, thus performing the Akiyama procedure without damaging the organs and structures of the neck, but the cervical phase took me longer as an operative time. On the seventh postoperative day, I do an oral contrast test (see Figures 8.1 and 8.2). On the 18th day, the patient is discharged from the hospital in good health.

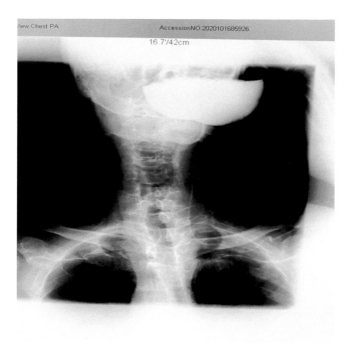

Figure 8.1 Radiologic examination with oral contrast.

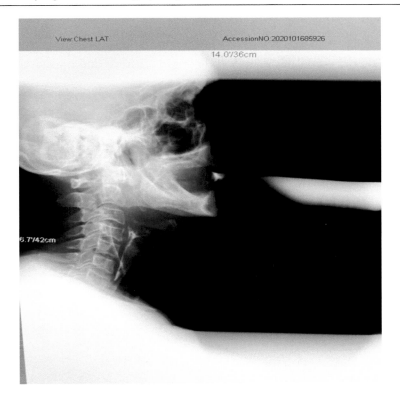

Figure 8.2 Lateral view of another radiologic examination with oral contrast.

8.3   PREOPERATIVE CARE

Patients with carcinoma of the esophagus are malnourished, with depletion of fat and protein reserves as well as dehydrated, this is a consequence of prolonged stenosis.

Before performing the operation of resection of the esophagus, this malnourishment must be corrected, and we do it by placing a jejunostomy.

The patient's respiratory preparation is necessary to avoid pulmonary complications that may be caused by the long duration of the intervention or thoracotomy. In case the patient is a smoker, smoking is stopped as soon as possible, and the application of bronchial hygiene therapy is also important:

- Various exercises for deep breathing.
- Coughing.

- Occasional inflation of balloons to effectively use the diaphragm and improve the strength of the respiratory muscles.

Even in patients who are in good condition and present a low complication rate, they should definitely undergo positive pressure breathing therapy with or without a bronchodilator.

A prophylactic dose of antibiotics should be applied two or three days before the intervention, as well as bowel cleansing with a laxative.

Systemic disorders are usually found in patients with esophageal carcinoma, as they are elderly. Of all the systems, that of hepatic insufficiency should be looked at carefully and should definitely be corrected, otherwise the case should not be operated on.

It is also important to familiarize the patient with the hospital, his familiarity with the operative technique, with the postoperative environment, that is, with the intensive care unit to minimize fear.

It is vital to cooperate with the patient by explaining:

- The duration of the intervention.
- Postoperative pains.
- The long period that they will not consume by mouth.
- The general discomfort.
- Administration of oxygen.

8.3.1   Intraoperative Attention

During the intervention, it is necessary to correct hypovolemia and hypoproteinemia, but we must be careful of overhydration. Human albumin, plasma, and blood should be administered with caution.

8.4   POSTOPERATIVE CARE

Patient preparation for surgical intervention and postoperative care.

A condition for a successful result in esophageal surgery is an adequate assessment of the general condition of the patient before the operation as well as an assessment of the risk that comes after the surgical act.

Factors related to the patient that negatively affect the postoperative result are:

- Age of the patient.
- Maldigestion as a result of esophageal stenosis.
- Adjuvant chemotherapy increasing secondary immunosuppression.
- Concomitant diseases such as diabetes.

- Hypertension.
- Hepato-renal insufficiency.
- Chronic cardio-pulmonary diseases.

In general, after laparotomy and thoracotomy, breathing is restricted and alveolar ventilation decreases as a result of pain and elevation of the diaphragm. So basal collapse is inevitable, which leads to hypoxia. In addition to atelectasis, the cause of hypoxia can be:

- Pneumothorax.
- Hemothorax.
- Chylothorax.
- Pleural fluid.
- Pulmonary edema.
- Pneumonia, etc.

All these causes must be carefully corrected.

There are three main moments that we must pay attention to and that are unique after esophagectomy:

- Cleaning of saliva. After lymphatic drainage at the level of the trachea and main bronchi, ischemia of the main airways occurs. Their inflammation and increase in saliva occur. Generally, this is cleared by having the patient cough or aspirate with an aspirator or fibrobronchoscope. The addition of atelectasis occurs rarely, but is dangerous, so preventive measures should be taken.
- Patients are often elderly and hypoproteinemic. This requires strict postoperative monitoring of fluid balance, daily caloric intake, assessment of central venous pressure.
- On the other hand, overhydration accompanied by pronounced hypoalbumenemia leads to pulmonary edema in women, which can be difficult to correct. Therefore, we use small doses of diuretics.

In the first postoperative days, patients have a tendency to develop metabolic acidosis, the reabsorption of sodium and bicarbonate increases, as well as the output of chloride and hydrogen ions.

Correction of acidosis consists of increasing bicarbonate reserves and decreasing hyperkalemia.

From hypoventilation, carbon dioxide retention leads to respiratory acidosis. Administration of oxygen and assisted respiration is necessary.

Special attention should be paid to the cardiac system to correct blood pressure or cardiac rhythm disorders.

Pain management is imperative. Intravenous and subcutaneous analgesics and opiates are applied.

Acute psychosis often occur in these patients, therefore the psychological preparation of the patient before the intervention and the establishment of a good postoperative rapport are of great value.

Drains and surgical wounds are carefully checked. On the third postoperative day, we start feeding through the jejunostomy and on the eighth day after doing the gastrography test of the anastomosis, if we do not have anastomotic leakage, we start feeding by mouth.

Mobilizing the patient as soon as possible is also valuable in order to prevent various thrombosis and pulmonary embolism, helps in intestinal peristalsis, regulation of breathing, and extraction of pulmonary secretions.

Physiotherapy is also recommended after the removal of thoracic drains.

8.5 PREOPERATIVE RADIO-CHEMOTHERAPY

Before surgical resection, our patients diagnosed with esophageal cancer, as part of the treatment protocol, undergo an intervention in which a feeding jejunostomy is placed as well as neoadjuvant chemotherapy together with radiotherapy. For locally advanced esophageal tumors, the standard treatment is neoadjuvant chemo-radiotherapy based on the CROSS trial meta-analysis.

Neoadjuvant treatment has its positive effects demonstrated by the studies carried out, among which we mention the improvement of negative resection margins, a better response of the tumor to the treatment with reduction of the dimensions of the primary tumor, as well as improvement of life expectancy for each patient. On the other hand, other studies show that patients who underwent neoadjuvant chemo-radiotherapy before surgical intervention had more serious post-operative complications and a higher number of deaths related to tumor progression. No significant difference has been demonstrated between the two groups that undergo or not preoperative neoadjuvant therapy in terms of the mortality of these patients in meta-analyses or studies with a large number of patients, being considered statistically non-significant.

The treatment protocol followed in collaboration with the Oncology Department at the Mother Teresa University Hospital Center for esophageal cancer is as follows:

Patients receive a combination of 3-Dimensional Conformal Radiotherapy (3DCRT) and Intensity Modulated Radiotherapy (IMRT) with a total radiation dose of 45 Gy, delivered at a rate of 1.8 Gy per fraction (see Figures 8.3 and 8.4).

For patients with squamous cell tumors of the esophagus, the radiation therapy is combined with weekly administrations of cisplatin at a dosage of 30 mg/m2. In cases of esophageal adenocarcinoma, capecitabine is administered at a dosage of 800 mg/m2.

During neoadjuvant therapy, patients are positioned supine under CT guidance. Prior to each cycle of therapy, patients should have an empty stomach for at least three to four hours.

Gross tumor volume (GTVt) is calculated for the primary tumor, and GTVn is determined for metastatic lymph nodes.

The clinical target volume (CTV) is established based on consensus guidelines from the bibliography. For squamous cell carcinoma, CTV extends 3 cm beyond the tumor dimensions in all directions, while for esophageal adenocarcinoma, it extends 5 cm proximally and distally, with a radial extension of 0.5–1 cm.

The planning target volume (PTV) is calculated by adding 1–2 cm to CTV in the proximal and distal directions and 0.5–1 cm radially.

This treatment regimen aims to effectively manage esophageal cancer and is based on established guidelines and protocols. The response of the patients to the treatment is evaluated up to the fourth week after radiotherapy, through CT scan and fibro-gastroscopy. Post-surgical neoadjuvant therapy is also planned for each patient.

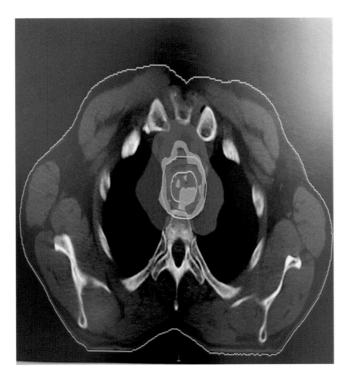

Figure 8.3 CT Image of IMRT—Oncological Department QSUT.

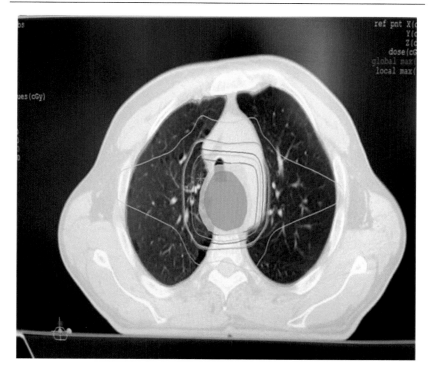

Figure 8.4 CT axial image of 3DCRT—Oncology Department QSUT.

Locally advanced squamous cell carcinoma located in the superior esophagus is treated with IMRT. CT image of IMRT shows the dispersion of 100%, 95%, and 50% of the administered dose.

Locally advanced squamous cell carcinoma of the medial portion of esophagus treated with 3DCRT. The CT axial image of 3DCRT shows the isodose dispersion.

In conclusion, our strategy is a combined treatment protocol of neoadjuvant therapy and surgery according to the guidelines cited above.

Most patients with esophageal tumors are diagnosed at an advanced stage locally and surgical intervention remains the best option for treatment. Despite the improvements in surgical techniques and the consequent improvement in life expectancy for these patients, the prognosis of these patients continues to be poor. In order to improve life expectancy during these last years, various alternatives have been developed by establishing preoperative treatment protocols of chemotherapy or chemotherapy combined with radiotherapy. Precisely based on these studies, despite the non-significant number and data that do not conclusively prove the positive results, this is also the protocol followed at our center.

In principle, preoperative neoadjuvant therapy should reduce the size of the tumor and this translates into ease for the surgeon during surgical resection.

Immune suppression and nutritional deficiency are considered important side effects of preoperative chemotherapy which can cause complications such as infections, fistulas, and delayed wound healing. In addition to the above-mentioned risks, the use of combined radiotherapy and chemotherapy increases the postoperative risk of having hemorrhage, fibrosis, technical difficulties in performing the anastomosis due to edema and adhesions, as well as respiratory problems due to damage to the pulmonary parenchyma.

What I want to add is the fact that the more the patient benefits from neoadjuvant chemo-radiotherapy, the more difficulties and problems it brings for the surgeon during the intervention, as a result of the fibrosis created after neoadjuvant therapy, so I would call it "surgeon's suffering".

BIBLIOGRAPHY

Narsule CK, Montgomery MM, Fernando HC. Evidence-based review of the management of cancers of the gastroesophageal junction. Thorac Surg Clin. 2012;22:109.

Rice TW, Kelsen D, Blackstone EH, et al. Esophagus and esophagogastric junction. In: Amin MB, editor. AJCC cancer staging manual. 8th ed. Chicago: AJCC; 2017. p. 185. Corrected at 4th printing, 2018.

Wu AJ, Goodman KA. Clinical tools to predict outcomes in patients with esophageal cancer treated with definitive chemoradiation: Are we there yet? J Gastrointest Oncol. 2015;6:53.

Lin SH, Wang J, Allen PK, et al. A nomogram that predicts pathologic complete response to neoadjuvant chemoradiation also predicts survival outcomes after definitive chemoradiation for esophageal cancer. J Gastrointest Oncol. 2015;6:45.

Kim JY, Correa AM, Vaporciyan AA, et al. Does the timing of esophagectomy after chemoradiation affect outcome? Ann Thorac Surg. 2012;93:207.

Pinotti HW. Extrapleural approach to the esophagus through frenolaparatomy (1976) AMB Rev Assoc Med Bras. 22:57–60 Transhiatal and transthoracic (thoracoscopy and thoracotomy esophagectomy for squamous-cell carcinoma (2006), p. 78, 10th World congress of the International Society for Diseases of the Esopahgus, Adelaide.

Markar SR, Arya S, Karthikesalingam A. Technical factors that affect anastomotic integrity following esophagectomy: Systematic review and meta-analysis. Ann Surg Oncol. 2013;20:4274–81.

Huang HT, Wang F, Shen L. Clinical outcome of middle thoracic esophageal cancer with intrathoracic or cervical anastomosis. Thorac Cardiovasc Surg. 2015;63:328–34.

Runkel N, Walz M, Ketelhut M. [Abdominothoracic esophageal resection according to Ivor Lewis with intrathoracic anastomosis: standardized totally minimally invasive technique]. Chirurg. 2015 May;86(5):468–75. doi: 10.1007/s00104-014-2786-y. PMID: 24994588.

Dapri G, Himpens J, Cadière GB. Minimally invasive esophagectomy for cancer: Laparoscopic transhiatal procedure or thoracoscopy in prone position followed by laparoscopy? Surg Endosc. 2008 Apr;22(4):1060–9. doi: 10.1007/s00464-007-9697-7. Epub 2007 Dec 11. PMID: 18071806.

Nguyen NT, Roberts P, Follette DM, et al. Thoracoscopic and laparoscopic esophagectomy for benign and malignant disease: Lessons learned from 46 consecutive procedures. J Am Coll Surg. 2003 Dec;197(6):902–13. doi: 10.1016/j.jamcollsurg.2003.07.005. PMID: 14644277.

Bizekis C, Kent MS, Luketich JD. Buenaventura PO initial experience with minimally invasive Ivor Lewis esophagectomy. Ann Thorac Surg. 2006 Aug;82(2):402–6; discussion 406–7. doi: 10.1016/j.athoracsur.2006.02.052. PMID: 16863737.

Campos GM, Jablons D, Brown LM, et al. A safe and reproducible anastomotic technique for minimally invasive Ivor Lewis oesophagectomy: The circular-stapled anastomosis with the trans-oral anvil. Eur J Cardiothorac Surg. 2010 Jun;37(6):1421–6. doi: 10.1016/j.ejcts.2010.01.010. Epub 2010 Feb 12. PMID: 20153660.

Böttger T, Terzic A, Müller M. [Extent of lymphnode dissection with minimally invasive esophageal resection]. Zentralbl Chir. 2006 Dec;131(6):466–73. doi: 10.1055/s-2006-955449. PMID: 17206565.

Valmasoni M, Capovilla G, Pierobon ES, et al. A technical modification to the circular stapling anastomosis technique during minimally invasive Ivor Lewis procedure. J Laparoendosc Adv Surg Tech A. 2019 Dec;29(12):1585–91. doi: 10.1089/lap.2019.0461. Epub 2019 Oct 3. PMID: 31580751.

Chapter 9

Complications

Esophagectomy is one of the major and most expensive surgical procedures, as a result it is accompanied by various complications, some of which are fatal for the patient.

I am focusing on the most important complications and among the most problematic to solve.

9.1 ANASTOMOTIC FISTULAS

This is the most problematic complication in esophageal surgery, whose clinical manifestation and treatment are closely related to resection methods and esophageal reconstruction methods. An important role in the prevention and treatment of anastomotic fistulas is played by the performance of the surgeon, who must possess three qualities:

1) To be correct in choosing the right method of resection of the esophagus.
2) Have very good knowledge of anatomy, morbidity, and physiology of the esophagus.
3) To be skilled in the correct implementation of surgical techniques.

The surgeon must select the type of resection and the method of esophageal reconstruction based on the qualities of the patients and the respective tumors, but no surgical technique has the same profit for all patients. A strong armament in the hands of the surgeon is a good knowledge of the complications of this type of surgery, which are important not only for the prevention of anastomotic complications but also for choosing the right treatment method. Early detection of complications and their treatment are vital for the patient. In some patients, the anastomotic fistulas are small, the leaks are occult and without clinical signs. Their diagnosis

   DOI: 10.1201/9781003497547-9

is made by examination with oral contrast. These fistulas are resolved by not giving the patient food by mouth, increasing the daily caloric intake that the patient must receive through jejunostomy food, as well as parenterally. Also, if there are signs of infection, broad-spectrum antibiotics, proton pump inhibitors, and somatostatin are added to the therapy.

In fistulas that present clinical symptoms, their treatment depends on the level of the anastomosis and the amount of leakage. Patients with a larger flow of intrathoracic fistulas require a re-intervention by pulling the stomach stump into the abdomen and cervical esophagostomy. The mortality rate in these cases reaches 95%. The sooner the fistula is diagnosed and re-intervention performed, the more the mortality rate decreases. In cases where the Akiyama procedure has been applied, the fistula is easier to treat by opening the wound at the level of the neck.

9.2 ANASTOMOTIC STENOSES

Anastomotic stenoses lead to dysphagia, but post-operative dysphagia can result not only from anastomotic stenoses but also from functional dysphagia. Stenoses are the result of anastomotic fistulas. Post-operative functional dysphagia can be caused by subtotal esophagectomy, insufficiency of the swallowing muscles as a result of a short esophagus. During the cervical incision, the neck muscles can be lacerated, which weakens the swallowing muscles. Likewise, denervation of the esophagus leads to slowing of gastric emptying.

Early stenoses, unlike late ones, are benign. Late ones in most cases are recurrences. In order to give the correct name to these stenoses, scanning and endoscopic examination are recommended.

In cases of early stenoses, bougie sessions are performed, but in a good part of cases the stenoses are removed without the need for bougie. In functional stenosis, we should focus on swallowing training and increasing enteral nutrition.

9.3 REFLUX AND DUMPING SYNDROME

Clinical signs of reflux are vomiting, cough, recurrent laryngitis, the patient cannot lie down, and recurrent pneumonia.

Dumping syndrome is common in this type of surgery, with 7% to 8% experiencing moderate symptoms and 2% experiencing severe symptoms. The factors that lead to dumping syndrome are denervation, reduction of the stomach, devascularization, abnormal functioning of the pylorus, which cause the stomach to empty quickly. Dumping syndrome is improved by changing the eating style, which includes eating in small and frequent amounts, avoiding drinking large amounts of liquids immediately after meals, avoiding the consumption of sweet foods, using foods rich in protein and poor in fats, not consuming dairy products. In some cases, we can use prednisolone, verapamil, propranolol.

9.4   DELAYED EMPTYING OF THE STOMACH

Delayed gastric emptying is a common complication. This is due to the reduction in the volume of the stomach, the vagotomy also leads to a malfunction of the pyloric sphincter, which is accompanied by vomiting or rapid satiety of the patient.

Improvement came from the use of domperidone, metoclopramide, cisapride, and erythromycin.

9.5   CHYLOTHORAX

Chylothorax is a rare complication with a percentage of 3.2% to 4%, but its inadequate treatment can lead to the loss of the patient.

In cases where the chylothorax has a volume smaller than 250–300 ml in 24 hours, then it is called controlled and is continued conservatively. If there continues to be a loss of 450 ml or more in 24 hours, it is considered as a failed conservative approach and re-intervention is definitely required, neglecting this moment can be fatal for the patient.

9.6   HEMOTHORAX AND HEMOPERITONEUM

It is not a rare complication that requires special attention and based on the volume of losses it may require an immediate re-intervention of the patient.

BIBLIOGRAPHY

Bray F, et al. Global cancer statistics 2018: GLOBOCAN estimates of incidence and mortality worldwide for 36 cancers in 185 countries. CA Cancer J Clin. 2018;68(6):394–424.

Jemal A, et al. Global cancer statistics. CA Cancer J Clin. 2011;61(2):69–90.

Ferlay J, et al. Cancer incidence and mortality worldwide: Sources, methods and major patterns in GLOBOCAN 2012. Int J Cancer. 2015;136(5):E359–86.

Siegel RL, Miller KD, Jemal A. Cancer statistics, 2019. CA Cancer J Clin. 2019;69(1):7–34.

Zeng H, et al. Changing cancer survival in China during 2003–15: A pooled analysis of 17 population-based cancer registries. Lancet Glob Health. 2018;6(5):e555–67.

Chen W, et al. Cancer statistics in China, 2015. CA Cancer J Clin. 2016; 66(2):115–32.

Feng RM, et al. Current cancer situation in China: Good or bad news from the 2018 global Cancer statistics? Cancer Commun (Lond). 2019;39(1):22.

Enzinger PC, Mayer RJ. Esophageal cancer. N Engl J Med. 2003;349(23):2241–52.

Ronkainen J, et al. Prevalence of Barrett's esophagus in the general population: An endoscopic study. Gastroenterol. 2005;129(6):1825–31.

Cook MB, et al. Cigarette smoking and adenocarcinomas of the esophagus and esophagogastric junction: A pooled analysis from the international BEACON consortium. J Natl Cancer Inst. 2010;102(17):1344–53.

Kato H, et al. Surgical treatment for esophageal cancer. Current Issues Dig Surg. 2007;24(2):88–95.

Agostinis P, et al. Photodynamic therapy of cancer: An update. CA Cancer J Clin. 2011;61(4):250–81.

Ono S, et al. Long-term outcomes of endoscopic submucosal dissection for superficial esophageal squamous cell neoplasms. Gastrointest Endosc. 2009;70(5):860–6.

Rustgi AK, El-Serag HB. Esophageal carcinoma. N Engl J Med. 2014;371(26): 2499–509.

Chapter 10

Discussion and Conclusions

Nowadays, there is a remarkable improvement in the quality of life and increased life expectancy for patients with esophageal carcinoma worldwide. This is thanks to the standardized protocol and its precise implementation in relation to this systemic disease.

However, we must accept the fact that surgery is only one link of this systemic disease. In patients with distant metastases, esophagectomy surgery has no benefit, and is contraindicated. There are patients in whom the location of the carcinoma is completely resectable, but clinically the patient does not benefit from surgery.

Clinics and surgery are two different but closely related aspects. With the development the diagnostic methods for esophageal carcinoma have received nowadays, I think it is easier for the surgeon to devise a clear plan regarding the esophageal surgery before the intervention.

However, in quite a few cases, it is not possible to detect small metastases. Therefore, the management of esophageal carcinoma is closely related to radio-chemotherapy, that is, multidisciplinary.

The prognosis of esophageal carcinoma surgery is related to the type of carcinoma itself. Extensive carcinomas with a deep infiltration have a very poor prognosis compared to more superficial carcinomas. However, to measure the prognosis is not easy.

I have had patients with short survival, in all these cases, in the biopsy report, identified lymph node and vascular involvement in various stations, that is, a high degree of malignancy. The surgeon would feel comfortable if the degree of malignancy for each patient were determined in advance, which is not possible. But lymphatic drainage is useful and necessary, as radiotherapy, immuno-cytotoxic chemotherapy also help the patient. There is still debate about the advantages and disadvantages of lymphatic curage.

But can a radical lymphatic curettage always be achieved?

Despite the fact that the main task for us surgeons is the complete lymphatic curettage, this is not always achieved due to the very fact of the

DOI: 10.1201/9781003497547-10

anatomical construction of the esophagus. In esophageal tumors, lymphatic drainage is easy and complete in the lower thoracic and abdominal cavity. The difficulty is encountered in the superior mediastinum and in the cervical part as the structures themselves are complicated and difficult to treat properly.

In order to have the best possible field of action for thoracic and cervical lymphatic drainage, many surgical variants have been described, but none of them are perfect and controversies continue about this. I think that the right thoracotomy and the left cervical opening is more optimal, I also admit that I cannot achieve a complete, that is, radical, lymphatic curettage in all cases.

10.1 CONTAMINATION OF THE OPERATIVE FIELD DURING LYMPHATIC DRAINAGE

The lymphatic vessels are of different diameters and during the curettage the small vessels are damaged and flow into the operative field, creating the possibility of the spread of cancer cells in the field.

Usually, we cut and tie the vessels with a large diameter, we cauterize the small ones, reducing the possibility of spreading neoplastic cells. The more delicately we treat the tissues, the more we reduce the risk of implantation of malignant cells in the operating field.

How does lymphatic drainage increase mortality?

Wide and radical curettage has its own risks, as it is performed in difficult and delicate regions such as the superior mediastinum and the cervical region, so we must be prudent. In the chest we can damage the trachea, bronchi, carina, laryngeal nerves which are not easy complications.

However, we have zero intraoperative mortality so far, curage is necessary, but each patient must be assessed before the intervention individually for the complexity it presents and a strategy created for the type of intervention we will perform. In case of lymph nodes involvement where curettage is not performed, regardless of esophagectomy, the operation is palliative, and the life expectancy of the patients is short. In fact, many patients come to us even now in advanced stages.

10.2 CASE PRESENTATION

A 70-year-old patient presents to the service with signs of severe dysphagia, drastic weight loss. Fibro-gastroscopy showed squamous carcinoma. A thoracoabdominal scan and magnetic resonance showed no distant metastases. Under these conditions, we implemented the protocol: the patient was placed with a nutritional jejunostomy and performed complete radiotherapy for 28 days as well as four chemotherapy sessions. Forty days after the end of radio-chemotherapy, the patient is re-hospitalized in the clinic to perform the esophagectomy. From the scanning examination and resonance now results with hepatic metastasis. The patient is very weary at the moment. Under these conditions, the case was considered inoperable, no intervention was made. Our question is, why does the patient metastasize under radio-chemotherapy? After reviewing the scanner and resonance again before placing the jejunostomy, I think we made a mistake in this case, the strategy used was not adequate. We ought to have the esophagus resected and then perform the radio-chemotherapy.

We should not always be strict in applying the oncological protocol in cases with carcinoma of the esophagus, but we should "get out of line", making exceptions based on the patient's clinical situation and our main goal is to improve the patient's life.

Although surgery remains the treatment of choice for esophageal carcinoma, there is much debate about the treatment route of choice: thoracotomy or transhiatal.

Both of these routes have their advantages and disadvantages. In transhiatal treatment, the advantages are the shorter duration of the intervention, avoiding thoracotomy, minimizing pulmonary complications, reducing the risk of mediastinitis, and minimizing postoperative pain. But I think that compared to thoracotomy in the transhiatal approach for cases of carcinoma in the middle and upper one-third, the lack of visualization of the tumor potentially endangers the oncological safety of the intervention, since lymphatic drainage is not performed radically, the recurrent nerve, trachea can be damaged, etc. However, the treatment course remains in the surgeon's preference, choosing a path in which they are sure, as the confidence and performance of the surgeon is life for the patient.

10.3   THE CARE WE MUST HAVE IN THE RETROSTERNAL PHASE

During the creation of the retrosternal tunnel, we must expand it as much as possible, so that the surgeon's forearm can enter. This dilation of the tunnel is done under its direct visualization and reduces the pressure exerted by both the left and right lungs on the gastric tube by increasing its blood supply.

The sternothyroid muscle posterior to the sternum must be partially cut to widen the upper opening of the retrosternal tunnel. This reduces the pressure on the stomach during muscle contraction, as a result the blood flow increases in the fundus of the stomach and at the level of the anastomosis. It also reduces the pressure at the anastomosis level.

The gastric tube should have a width of 3.5–4 cm, since the wider the tube, the better its upper part is supplied with blood through the micro-vascular system.

Fixing the tube to the tissues around the neck and at the level of the diaphragm helps prevent torsion.

All these affect the reduction of the risk of fistulas of cervical anastomosis.

10.4   THE ROLE OF JEJUNOSTOMY IN PATIENTS WITH ESOPHAGEAL CARCINOMA

Personally, I have used jejunostomy in 99% of cases, where in most cases I have placed it before the patient performs radio-chemotherapy and in a small number of cases I have used it during esophageal resection. Jejunostomy placement is at the surgeon's discretion. I started on the third post-operative day, both to promote peristalsis and to increase the patient's protein caloric intake, which is so necessary in this neoplastic pathology and the high aggression presented by this type of intervention, that is, esophagectomy.

It is also of great value in cases where we have leakage from the esophagogastric anastomosis, since through feeding from the jejunostomy we keep the necessary calories of the patient at optimal levels, so it gives a great help in the efforts we make for the conservative solution of esophagogastric fistulas.

There are different opinions regarding the routine placement of a feeding jejunostomy in esophageal resections, I personally would call its placement as "surgeon's peace of mind", regardless of whether it will work or not.

10.5   ESOPHAGEAL RESECTION MARGINS

We must pay great attention to the level of the esophagus resected, based on the tumor biopsy.

In the case of adenocarcinomas, the cutting level is sufficient up to 3 cm above the tumor, but in the case of squamous cell carcinomas, this cutting level of the esophagus must be above 5–7 cm to eliminate as much as possible seeding by neoplastic cells that are not evident with the naked eye. Some authors extend these margins to 10 cm.

Based on this fact, despite the fact that anatomically the esophagus is divided into three parts, I think and put it up for discussion, that surgically the esophagus is divided into two parts:

1) The lower part where the Ivor-Lewis procedure should be performed.
2) The middle and upper parts are taken together where the Akiyama or McKeown procedure should be performed.

A squamous cell carcinoma located in the middle one-third of the esophagus, respecting a resection distance of up to 7 cm leads to the realization of the eso-gastric anastomosis in the upper one-third of the esophagus and its intrathoracic implementation is done under difficult technical conditions, compared to cervical anastomosis where the surgeon feels more comfortable.

The difficult technical conditions for the realization of eso-gastric anastomosis constitute one of the factors that increase the risk of anastomotic fistulas. In the same way, the management of cervical eso-gastric fistulas is easier than intrathoracic. Therefore, I think about this division from the surgical point of view of the esophagus.

Why do I prefer the Akiyama procedure compared to McKeown?
Why do I prefer the stomach to replace the esophagus and not the colon?

In the first place, I prefer the gastric tube as an option to replace the esophagus, as it is more physiological in terms of the structure of the gastro-intestinal tract itself.

There are three ways to place the gastric tube: parasternal, retrosternal, and posterior mediastinal.

I prefer the retrosternal route, that is, the Akiyama procedure, as:

1) This significantly reduces gastro-oesophageal reflux.
2) Significantly reduces the risk of eso-gastric anastomotic fistulas and makes it easier to manage these fistulas when they occur.
3) Reduces the tendency to gastrectasia.
4) With the retrosternal route, we create a new route of the digestive tract excluding the entire area of the posterior mediastinum where the tumor was located together with the tissue around it.
5) In cases where postoperative radiotherapy will be performed, the retrosternal route ensures that the stomach and eso-gastric anastomosis are not damaged by radiotherapy.
6) Reduces the risk of pneumonia.

Whereas the disadvantage of the Akiyama procedure is the bad sensation of the patients when swallowing in the first postoperative weeks, then everything normalizes.

Thank you for your attention to this modest monograph.

I continue to be of the opinion that it is the most difficult surgery with many unexpected events, but the surgeon feels proud when they sally forth into the unattainable peaks whether they reach them or not.

Esophageal cancer is one of the most aggressive tumors of the human body, and as a surgery it is the toughest and most exhausting for the surgeon. However, what pushes the surgeon to deal with this type of surgery is the fulfillment of the only desire of the patient, the desire to eat. All instincts that are born with the human wane and disappear with age, but the feeding instinct accompanies him from birth until his parting from life.

To be continued . . .

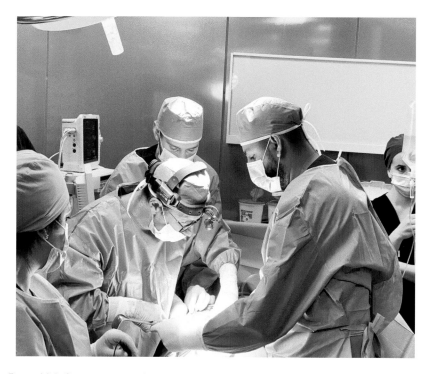

Figure 10.1 Surgeons team during the procedure.

BIBLIOGRAPHY

Sjoquist KM, Smithers BM, Burmeister BH. Survival after neoadjuvant chemotherapy or chemoradiotherapy for resectable oesophageal carcinoma: An updated meta-analysis. Lancet Oncol. 2011;11:671–91.

Pennathur A, Luketich JD, Ward J, et al. Long-term results of a phase II trial of neoadjuvant chemotherapy followed by esophagectomy for locally advanced esophageal neoplasm. Ann Thorac Surg. 2008 Jun;86(6):1930–5; discussion 1935–7. doi: 10.1016/j.athoracsur.2008.01.097. PMID: 18498697.

Clavien PA, de Oliveira ML, Barkun J, et al. The Clavien-Dindo classification of surgical complications: Five-year experience. Ann Surg. 2009;251:186–95.

Kumagai K, Rouvelas I, Tsai JA, et al. Meta-analysis of postoperative morbidity and perioperative mortality in patients receiving neoadjuvant chemotherapy or chemoradiotherapy for resectable oesophageal and gastro-oesophageal junctional cancers. Br J Surg. 2014;101:325–37.

Al-Sukhni E, Attwood K, Gabriel E, et al. No survival difference with neoadjuvant chemoradiotherapy compared with chemotherapy in resectable esophageal and gastroesophageal junction adenocarcinoma: Results from the national cancer data base. J Am Coll Surg 2016;226:785–91.e1.

Luu TD, Force SD, Gaur P, et al. Neoadjuvant chemoradiation versus chemotherapy for patients undergoing esophagectomy for esophageal cancer. Ann Thorac Surg. 2008;85:1217–24; discussion 1225–4.

Abraham JW, Walter DT, Chang RB, et al. Expert consensus contouring guidelines for IMRT in esophageal and gastroesophageal junction 13cancer. Int J Radiat Oncol Biol Phys. 2015 July 15;92(4):914–22. doi:10.1026/.

Khan FM, Gerbi BJ. Treatment planning in radiation oncology. 3rd ed. Philadelphia, PA: Lippincott William & Wilkins/Wolters Kluwer; 2012.

Donington JS, Deschamps C, Nichols FC III, Miller DL, Allen MS, Pairolero PC. Preoperative chemoradiation therapy does not improve early survival after esophagectomy for patients with clinical stage III adenocarcinoma the esophagus. Ann Thorac Surg. 2004;76:1196–9.

Lin FC, Ferguson MK, Durkin AE. Induction therapy does not increase surgical morbidity after esophagectomy for cancer. Ann Thorac Surg. 2004;77:1793–8.

Lee CH, Lee JM, Wu DC, et al. Carcinogenetic impact of alcohol intake on squamous cell carcinoma risk of the oesophagus in relation to tobacco smoking. Eur J Cancer 2007;44:1288–99.

Umar SB, Fleischer DE, Lee JM. Esophageal cancer: Epidemiology, pathogenesis and prevention. Nat Clin Pract Gastroenterol Hepatol 2008;5:537–42.

Barrios E, De Stefani E, Fierro L. Black (air-cured) and blond (flue-cured) tobacco and cancer risk. III: Oesophageal cancer. Eur J Cancer 1993;29A:764–768.

Kristal A, Vaughan TL, Davis S, et al. Obesity, alcohol, and tobacco as risk factors for cancers of the esophagus and gastric cardia: Adenocarcinoma versus squamous cell carcinoma. Cancer Epidemiol Biomarkers Prev 1995;4:86–93.

Silverman D, Brown LM, Hoover R, et al. Excess incidence of squamous cell esophageal cancer among US Black men: Role of social class and other risk factors. Am J Epidemiol. 2001;153:115–23.

Abnet CC, Mark SD. Prospective study of tooth loss and incident esophageal and gastric cancers in China. Cancer Causes Control 2001;12:848–57.

Yang SJ, Wang HY, et al. Genetic polymorphisms of ADH2 and ALDH2 association with esophageal cancer risk in southwest China. World J Gastroenterol 2007;13:576.

Risk JM, Garde J, et al. The tylosis esophageal cancer (TOC) locus: More than just a familial cancer gene. Dis Esophagus. 1999;12:178–9.

Poynton AR, O'Sullivan G. Carcinoma arising in familial Barrett's esophagus. Am J Gastroenterol. 1996;91:185.

Bollschweller, Holscher AH, et al. Prognostic differences between early squamous cell and adenocarcinoma of the esophagus. Dis esophagus. 1997;10:178–83.

The American Joint Committee on Cancer: The 7th edition of the AJCC cancer staging manual and the future of TNM Stephen B Edge. Carolyn C Compton n Surg Oncol 2010 Jun;17(6):1481–4.

Cameron AJ, Conio M, et al. Endoscopic treatment of high-grade dysplasia and early cancer in Barrett's esophagus. Review. Lancet Oncology. 2005:1–2.

Gossner L Ell C, Mat A, et al. Endoscopic mucosal resection of early cancer high-grade dysplasia in Barrett's esophagus. Gastroenterol. 2000:670–9.

Kanao H, Tanaka S. Clinical significance of type V pit pattern subclassification in determining the depth of invasion of colorectal neoplasms. World J Gastroenterol. 2008 Jan 14:211–2178.

Bonavina I, Incarbone R, Bona D, Peracchia A. Esofagectomy—it is not just mortality anymore: Standardized perioperative clinical pathways improve outcomes in patients with esophageal cancer. J Gastrointest Surg. 2007 Feb;14(1):13–6. doi: 10.1089/109264204322862298. PMID: 15035838.

Kunz S, Low DE, Schembre D, et al. Esofagectomy—it is not just mortality anymore: Standardized perioperative clinical pathways improve outcomes in patients with esophageal cancer. J Gastrointest Surg. 2007.

Orringer MB, Marshall B, Chang AC, et al. Two thousand transhiatal esophagectomies: Charging trends, lessons learned. Ann Surg. 2007 Sep;246(3):363–72; discussion 372–4. doi: 10.1097/SLA.0b013e31814697f2. PMID: 17717440; PMCID: PMC1959358.

Greenstein AJ, Litle VR, Swanson SJ, et al. Effect of the number of lymphnodes sampled on prospective survival of lymph node negative esophageal cancer. Cancer. 2008 Mar 15;112(6):1239–46. doi: 10.1002/cncr.23309. PMID: 18224663.

Coda S, Oda I, Saito Y. EMR and ESD for early gastrointestinal cancers. In: Conio M, Siersema PD, Repici A, et al. editors. Endoscopic Mucosal Resection. Oxford: Blackwell Publishing; 2008. p. 185–98.

Ronellenfitsch U, Schwarzbach M, Hofheitz R, et al. Preoperative Cheo(radio) therapy versus primary surgery for gastroesophageal adenocarcinoma: Systematic review with meta-analysis combining individual patient and aggregate data. Eur J Cancer. 2013 Oct;49(15):3149–58. doi: 10.1016/j.ejca.2013.05.029. Epub 2013 Jun 22. PMID: 23800671.

Li X, Zhao LJ, Liu NB, et al. Feasibility and efficacy of concurrent chemoradiotherapy in elderly patients with esophageal squamous carcinoma: A retrospective study of 116 cases from a single institution. Asian Pac J Cancer Prev. 2015;16(4):1463–9. doi: 10.7314/apjcp.2015.16.4.1463. PMID: 25743816.

Jenkinson AD, Lim J, Agrawl N, et al. Laparoscopic feeding jejunostomy in esophagogastric cancer. Surg Endosc. 2007. Evolué de l'oesophage thoracique. Anastomose oesogastrique au cou ou dans le thorax? Résultats tardifs d'une étude prospective "randomisée". Ann Chir. 1992;46:905–11.

Lam TCF, Fok M, Cheng SW, Wong J. Anastomotic complications after esophagectomy for cancer: A comparison of neck and chest anastomoses. J Thor Cardiovasc Surg. 1992;104:395–400.

Akiyama H, Tsurumaru M, Udagawa H, et al. Radical lymph node dissection for cancer of the thoracic oesophagus. Ann Surg. 1994;220:364–373.

Baba M, Aikou T, Yoshinaka H, et al. Long-term results of subtotal esophagectomy with three-field lymphadenectomy for carcinoma of the thoracic esophagus. Ann Surg. 1994;219:310–16.

Nishihira T, Hirayama K, Mori S. Aprospective randomized trial of extended cervical and superior mediastinal lymphadenectomy for carcinoma of the thoracic esophagus. Am J Surg. 1998;175:47–51.

Hayes N, Shaw IH, Raimes SA, et al. Comparison of conventional Lewis-Tanner two-stage oesophagectomy with the synchronous two-team approach. Br J Surg. 1995;82:95–7.

Triboulet JP, Mariette C, Chevalier D, et al. Surgical management of carcinoma of the hypopharynx and cervical esophagus: Analysis of 209 cases. Arch Surg. 2001;136:1164–70.

Couraud L, Velly JF, Clerc P, et al. Experience of partial oesophagectomy in surgical treatment of lower and middle thoracic oesophageal cancer. From a follow-up of 366 cases. Eur J Cardiothorac Surg. 1989;3(2):99–103; discussion 104. doi: 10.1016/1010-7940(89)90085-7. PMID: 248334.

Cense HA, van Eijck CH, Tilanus HW. New insights in the lymphatic spread of oesophageal cancer and its implications for the extent of surgical resection. Best Pract Res Clin Gastroenterol. 2006;20(5):893–906. doi: 10.1016/j.bpg.2006.03.010. PMID: 16997168.

Bîrlă R, Iosif C, Mocanu A, et al. [Long-term survival after eso-gastrectomy for esophagogastric junction adenocarcinoma–prospective study]. Chirurgia (Bucur). 2008 Nov–Dec;103(6):635–42. PMID: 19274907 Romanian.

Pedrazzani C, Pasini F, Giacopuzzi S, et al. [Surgical treatment of gasto-esophageal junction adenocarcinoma: Long-term results of a single Italian centre]. G Chir. 2004 Oct;25(10):325–33. PMID: 15756954.

Stein HJ, Feith M, Siewert JR. Individualized surgical strategies for cancer of the esophagogastric junction. Ann Chir Gynaecol. 2000;89(3):191–8. PMID: 11079787.

Feith M, Stein HJ, Siewert JR. Adenocarcinoma of the esophagogastric junction: Surgical therapy based on 1602 consecutive resected patients. Surg Oncol Clin N Am. 2006 Oct;15(4):751–64. doi: 10.1016/j.soc.2006.07.015. PMID: 17030271.

Rüdiger Siewert J, Feith M, Werner M, et al. Adenocarcinoma of the esophagogastric junction: Results of surgical therapy based on anatomical/topographic classification in 1,002 consecutive patients. Ann Surg. 2000 Sep;232(3):353–61. doi: 10.1097/00000658-200009000-00007. PMID: 10973385.

Mönig SP, Schröder W, Beckurts KT, et al. Classification, diagnosis and surgical treatment of carcinomas of the gastroesophageal junction. Hepatogastroenterology. 2001 Sep–Oct;48(41):1231–7. PMID: 11677937.

Bai JG, Lv Y, Dang CX. Adenocarcinoma of the Esophagogastric Junction in China according to Siewert's classification. Jpn J Clin Oncol. 2006 Jun;36(6):364–7. doi: 10.1093/jjco/hyl042. Epub 2006 Jun 9. PMID: 16766566.

McManus K, Anikin V, McGuigan J. Total thoracic oesophagectomy for oesophageal carcinoma: Has it been worth it? Eur J Cardiothorac Surg. 1999 Sep;16(3):261–5. doi: 10.1016/s1010-7940(99)00223-7. PMID: 10554840.

Maher M, Ali A, Qureshi H, et al. Transhiatal oesophagectomy for carcinoma oesophagus. Early experience. J Pak Med Assoc. 1991 Jun;41(6):129–31. PMID: 1895496.

Rindani R, Martin CJ, Cox MR. Transhiatal versus Ivor-Lewis oesophagectomy: Is there a difference? Aust N Z J Surg. 1999 Mar;69(3):187–94. doi: 10.1046/j.1440-1622.1999.01520.x. PMID: 10075357.

Omloo JM, Lagarde SM, Hulscher JB, et al. Extended transthoracic resection compared with limited transhiatal resection for adenocarcinoma of the mid/distal esophagus: Five-year survival of a randomized clinical trial. Ann Surg. 2007 Dec;246(6):992–1000; discussion 1000–1. doi: 10.1097/SLA.0b013e31815c4037. PMID: 18043101.

Peracchia A, Bonavina L, Via A, et al. Current trends in the surgical treatment of esophageal and cardia adenocarcinoma. J Exp Clin Cancer Res. 1999 Sep;18(3):289–94. PMID: 10606171.

Walther B, Johansson J, Johnsson F, et al. Cervical or thoracic anastomosis after esophageal resection and gastric tube reconstruction: A prospective randomized trial comparing sutured neck anastomosis with stapled intrathoracic anastomosis. Ann Surg. 2003 Dec;238(6):803–12; discussion 812–4. doi: 10.1097/01.sla.0000098624.04100.b1. PMID: 14631217.

Fok M, Wong J. Cancer of the oesophagus and gastric cardia: Standard oesophagectomy and anastomotic technique. Ann Chir Gynaecol. 1995;84(2):179–83. PMID: 7574378.

Kimose HH, Lund O, Hasenkam JM, et al. Independent predictors of operative mortality and postoperative complications in surgically treated carcinomas of the oesophagus and cardia–is the aggressive surgical approach worthwhile? Acta Chir Scand. 1990 May;156(5):373–82. PMID: 1693462.

Svanes K, Stangeland L, Viste A, et al. Morbidity, ability to swallow, and survival, after oesophagectomy for cancer of the oesophagus and cardia. Eur J Surg. 1995 Sep;161(9):669–75. PMID: 8541426.

Jensen BM, Andersen KB. [Surgical treatment of cancer of the esophagus and cardia]. Ugeskr Laeger. 1998 Jul 27;160(31):4531–3. PMID: 9700310.

Sabanathan S, Eng J. Left thoracotomy approach for resection of carcinoma of the oesophagus and cardia. Ann Ital Chir. 1992 Jan–Feb;63(1):25–31. PMID: 1605442.

Kakeji Y, Takahashi A, Hasegawa H, et al. Surgical outcomes in gastroenterological surgery in Japan: Report of the National Clinical Database 2011–2018. Ann Gastroenterol Surg. 2020;4:250–74.

Takeuchi H, Miyata H, Gotoh M, et al. A risk model for esophagectomy using data of 5354 patients included in a Japanese nationwide web-based database. Ann Surg. 2014;260:259–66.

Chevallay M, Jung M, Chon SH, et al. Esophageal cancer surgery: Review of complications and their management. Ann N Y Acad Sci. 2020;1482:146–62.

Markar S, Gronnier C, Duhamel A, et al. The impact of severe anastomotic leak on long-term survival and cancer recurrence after surgical resection for esophageal malignancy. Ann Surg. 2015;262:972–80.

Jansen SM, de Bruin DM, van Berge Henegouwen MI, et al. Optical techniques for perfusion monitoring of the gastric tube after esophagectomy: A review of technologies and thresholds. Dis Esophagus. 2018;1:31.

Brinkmann S, Chang DH, Kuhr K, et al. Stenosis of the celiac trunk is associated with anastomotic leak after Ivor-Lewis esophagectomy. Dis Esophagus. 2019;1:32.

Tsunoda S, Obama K, Hisamori S, et al. Lower incidence of postoperative pulmonary complications following robot-assisted minimally invasive esophagectomy for esophageal cancer: propensity score-matched comparison to conventional minimally invasive esophagectomy. Ann Surg Oncol. 2021;28:639–47.

Lainas P, Fuks D, Gaujoux S, et al. Preoperative imaging and prediction of oesophageal conduit necrosis after oesophagectomy for cancer. Br J Surg. 2017;104:1346–54.

Robba C, Cardim D, Sekhon M, et al. Transcranial doppler: A stethoscope for the brain-neurocritical care use. J Neurosci Res. 2018;96:720–30.

Noshiro H, Urata M, Ikeda O, et al. Invasive esophagectomy. Surgery. 2013;154:604–10.

Kim EN, Lamb K, Relles D, et al. Median arcuate ligament syndrome-review of this rare disease. JAMA Surg. 2016;151:471–7.

Horton KM, Talamini MA, Fishman EK. Median arcuate ligament syndrome: Evaluation with CT angiography. Radiographics. 2005;25:1177–82.

Liebermann-Meffert DM, Meier R, Siewert JR. Vascular anatomy of the gastric tube used for esophageal reconstruction. Ann Thorac Surg. 1992;54:1110–5.

Lammerts RGM, van Det MJ, Geelkerken RH, et al. Risk-assessment of esophageal surgery: Diagnosis and treatment of celiac trunk stenosis. Thorac Cardiovasc Surg Rep. 2018;7:e21–3.

Kassis ES, Kosinski AS, Ross P Jr, et al. Predictors of anastomotic leak after esophagectomy: An analysis of the society of thoracic surgeons general thoracic database. Ann Thorac Surg 2013;96:1919–26.

Markar SR, Arya S, Karthikesalingam A, et al. Technical factors that affect anastomotic integrity following esophagectomy: systematic review and meta-analysis. Ann Surg Oncol. 2013;20:4274–81.

Schmidt HM, Gisbertz SS, Moons J, et al. Denning benchmarks for transthoracic esophagectomy: A multicenter analysis of total minimally invasive esophagectomy in low risk patients. Ann Surg 2017;266:814–21.

Huang HT, Wang F, Shen L, et al. Clinical outcome of middle thoracic esophageal cancer with intrathoracic or cervical anastomosis. Thorac Cardiovasc Surg. 2015 Jun;63(4):328–34. doi: 10.1055/s-0034-1371509. Epub 2014 Apr 8. PMID: 24715527.

Wormald JC, Bennett J, van Leuven M, et al. Does the site of anastomosis for esophagectomy affect long-term quality of life? Dis Esophagus. 2016;29:93–8.

Akiyama S, Ito S, Sekiguchi H, et al. Preoperative embolization of gastric arteries for esophageal cancer. Surgery 1996;120:542–6.

D'Amico TA. Outcomes after surgery for esophageal cancer. Gastrointest Cancer Res. 2007;1:188.

Hirst J, Smithers BM, Gotley DC, et al. Defining cure for esophageal cancer: analysis of actual 5-year survivors following esophagectomy. Ann Surg Oncol. 2011;18:1766.

Markar SR, Karthikesalingam A, Thrumurthy S, et al. Volume-outcome relationship in surgery for esophageal malignancy: systematic review and meta-analysis 2000–2011. J Gastrointest Surg. 2012;16:1055.

Narsule CK, Montgomery MM, Fernando HC. Evidence-based review of the management of cancers of the gastroesophageal junction. Thorac Surg Clin. 2012;22:109.

Rice TW, Kelsen D, Blackstone EH, et al. Esophagus and esophagogastric junction. In: Amin MB, editors. AJCC cancer staging manual. 8th ed. Chicago: AJCC; 2017. p. 185. Corrected at 4th printing, 2018.

Wu AJ, Goodman KA. Clinical tools to predict outcomes in patients with esophageal cancer treated with definitive chemoradiation: are we there yet? J Gastrointest Oncol. 2015;6:53.

Lin SH, Wang J, Allen PK, et al. A nomogram that predicts pathologic complete response to neoadjuvant chemoradiation also predicts survival outcomes after definitive chemoradiation for esophageal cancer. J Gastrointest Oncol. 2015;6:45.

Kim JY, Correa AM, Vaporciyan AA, et al. Does the timing of esophagectomy after chemoradiation affect outcome? Ann Thorac Surg. 2012;93:207.

Pinotti HW. Extrapleural approach to the esophagus through frenolaparatomy. AMB Rev Assoc Med Bras. 1976;22:57–60. Transhiatal and transthoracic (thoracoscopy and thoracotomy esophagectomy for squamous-cell carcinoma (2006), p. 78, 10th World congress of the International Society for Diseases of the Esopahgus, Adelaide. 10th World congress of the International Society for Diseases of the Esopahgus Congress Handbook

Markar SR, Arya S, Karthikesalingam A. Technical factors that affect anastomotic integrity following esophagectomy: Systematic review and meta-analysis. Ann Surg Oncol. 2013;20:4274–81.

Huang HT, Wang F, Shen L. Clinical outcome of middle thoracic esophageal cancer with intrathoracic or cervical anastomosis. Thorac Cardiovasc Surg. 2015;63:328–34.

Runkel N, Walz M, Ketelhut M. [Abdominothoracic esophageal resection according to Ivor Lewis with intrathoracic anastomosis: Standardized totally minimally invasive technique]. Chirurg. 2015 May;86(5):468–75. doi: 10.1007/s00104-014-2786-y. PMID: 24994588.

Dapri G, Himpens J, Cadière GB. Minimally invasive esophagectomy for cancer: Laparoscopic transhiatal procedure or thoracoscopy in prone position followed by laparoscopy? Surg Endosc. 2008 Apr;22(4):1060–9. doi: 10.1007/s00464-007-9697-7. Epub 2007 Dec 11. PMID: 18071806.

Nguyen NT, Roberts P, Follette DM, et al. Thoracoscopic and laparoscopic esophagectomy for benign and malignant disease: Lessons learned from 46 consecutive procedures. J Am Coll Surg. 2003 Dec;197(6):902–13. doi: 10.1016/j.jamcollsurg.2003.07.005. PMID: 14644277.

Bizekis C, Kent MS, Luketich JD. Buenaventura PO initial experience with minimally invasive Ivor Lewis esophagectomy. Ann Thorac Surg. 2006 Aug;82(2):402–6; discussion 406–7. doi: 10.1016/j.athoracsur.2006.02.052. PMID: 16863737.

Campos GM, Jablons D, Brown LM, et al. A safe and reproducible anastomotic technique for minimally invasive Ivor Lewis oesophagectomy: The circular-stapled anastomosis with the trans-oral anvil. Eur J Cardiothorac Surg. 2010 Jun;37(6):1421–6. doi: 10.1016/j.ejcts.2010.01.010. Epub 2010 Feb 12. PMID: 20153660.

Böttger T, Terzic A, Müller M. [Extent of lymphnode dissection with minimally invasive esophageal resection]. Zentralbl Chir. 2006 Dec;131(6):466–73. doi: 10.1055/s-2006-955449. PMID: 17206565.

Valmasoni M, Capovilla G, Pierobon ES, et al. A technical modification to the circular stapling anastomosis technique during minimally invasive ivor lewis procedure. J Laparoendosc Adv Surg Tech A. 2019 Dec;29(12):1585–1591. doi: 10.1089/lap.2019.0461. Epub 2019 Oct 3. PMID: 31580751.

He F, Wang J, Liu L, et al. Esophageal cancer: Trends in incidence and mortality in China from 2005 to 2015. Cancer Med. 2021;10(5):1839–47. doi: 10.1002/cam4.3647.

Sung H, Ferlay J, Siegel RL, et al. Global cancer statistics 2020: Globocan estimates of incidence and mortality worldwide for 36 cancers in 185 countries. CA: Cancer J Clin. 2021;71(3):209–49. doi: 10.3322/caac.21660.

Abnet CC, Arnold M, Wei WQ. Epidemiology of esophageal squamous cell carcinoma. Gastroenterol. 2018;154(2):360–73. doi: 10.1053/j.gastro.2017.08.023.

Ajani JA, D'Amico TA, Bentrem DJ, et al. Esophageal and esophagogastric junction cancers, version 2.2019, NCCN clinical practice guidelines in oncology. J Natl Compr Cancer Network JNCCN. 2019;17(7):855–83. doi: 10.6004/jnccn.2019.0033.

Yanagimoto Y, Kurokawa Y, Doki Y, et al. Surgical and perioperative treatment strategy for resectable esophagogastric junction cancer. Japanese J Clin Oncol. 2022;52(5):417–24. doi: 10.1093/jjco/hyac019.

Yang H, Liu H, Chen Y, et al. Long-term efficacy of neoadjuvant chemoradiotherapy plus surgery for the treatment of locally advanced esophageal squamous cell carcinoma: The Neocrtec5010 randomized clinical trial. JAMA Surg. 2021;156(8):721–9. doi: 10.1001/jamasurg.2021.2373.

Li Z, Sun G, Sun G, et al. Various uses of Pd1/Pd-L1 inhibitor in oncology: Opportunities and challenges. Front Oncol. 2021;11:771335. doi: 10.3389/fonc.2021.77133.

Wang C, Sandhu J, Ouyang C, et al. Clinical response to immunotherapy targeting programmed cell death receptor 1/Programmed cell death ligand 1 in patients with treatment-resistant microsatellite stable colorectal cancer with and without liver metastases. JAMA Network Open. 2021;4(8):e2118416. doi: 10.1001/jamanetworkopen.2021.18416105.

Zhang W, Wang P, Pang Q. Immune checkpoint inhibitors for esophageal squamous cell carcinoma: A narrative review. Ann Trans Med. 2020;8(18):1193. doi: 10.21037/atm-20-462.

Qiu HB. Safety and efficacy of tislelizumab plus chemotherapy for first-line treatment of advanced esophageal squamous cell carcinoma and Gastric/Gastroesophageal junction adenocarcinoma. Thorac Cancer. 2020;11(12):3419–21. doi: 10.1111/1759-7714.13690.

Mamdani H, Schneider B, Perkins SM, et al. A phase ii trial of adjuvant durvalumab following trimodality therapy for locally advanced esophageal and gastroesophageal junction adenocarcinoma: A big ten cancer research consortium study. Front Oncol. 2021;11:736620. doi: 10.3389/fonc.2021.736620.

Ma J, Zhan C, Wang L, et al. The sweet approach is still worthwhile in modern esophagectomy. Ann Thorac Surg. 2014;97(5):1728–33. doi: 10.1016/j.athoracsur.2014.01.034.

Zheng Y, Li Y, Liu X, et al. Right compared with left thoracic approach esophagectomy for patients with middle esophageal squamous cell carcinoma. Front Oncol. 2020;10:536842. doi: 10.3389/fonc.2020.536842.

Voeten DM, Busweiler LAD, van der Werf LR, et al. Outcomes of esophagogastric cancer surgery during eight years of surgical auditing by the Dutch upper gastrointestinal cancer audit (Duca). Ann Surg. 2021;274(5):866–73.

Inada M, Nishimura Y, Ishikawa K, et al. Comparing the 7th and 8th editions of the American joint committee on Cancer/Union for international cancer control TNM staging system for esophageal squamous cell carcinoma treated by definitive radiotherapy. Esophagus Off J Japan Esophageal Soc. 2019;16(4):371–6.

Index